"In this impressive and highly readable book, Lloyd Sederer explores the science, the law, and the social reality of addiction. This is a needed and timely volume for those who are fighting addiction and for their families, as well as for all of us who live in a world increasingly riven by substance abuse."

—Andrew Solomon, *New York Times* bestselling author of *The Noonday Demon* and *Far from the Tree*

"In the United States, psychiatry has for too long had a very narrow and simplistic understanding of addiction—so it's really exciting to read a wise psychiatrist engaging deeply with this subject. This is a humane and intelligent book."

—Johann Hari, *New York Times* bestselling author of *Chasing the Scream: The First and Last Days of the War on Drugs*

"*The Addiction Solution* is a wise and humane book about one of our hardest problems—that of addiction and its consequences. Drawing on decades of clinical and policy experience, Dr. Sederer makes an important contribution to our understanding of this problem. I emerged from reading it with clarity about the bold steps we must take collectively to move beyond addiction, to create a healthier world, and I am grateful to Dr. Sederer for writing this book."

—Dr. Sandro Galea, MD, DrPH, Robert A. Knox professor and dean of the Boston University School of Public Health and former president of the Society for Epidemiologic Research

"Dr. Sederer writes with clarity and compassion, and suggests sensible and humane answers. This book is impressive, timely, and valuable."

—Lee Child, *New York Times* bestselling author of the Jack Reacher series

"Like Dr. Sederer's other works, this book is a pleasure to read. *The Addiction Solution* covers a complex and controversial subject in plain, jargon-free language. The book does more than inform: it offers solutions."

—Andrew Kolodny, MD, codirector, Opioid Policy Research Collaborative, Heller School for Social Policy and Management, Brandeis University

"Dr. Lloyd Sederer is one of the most informed and informative experts on mental health and addiction in this country. But more than that, he's a brilliant healer whose intellect is matched by his humanity. He's a sterling public servant and a terrific writer as well, and his new book on addictions is timely, important, and a *must-read* for anyone who cares about addiction and its impact on our lives, our families, and our society."

—John Fugelsang, host of *Tell Me Everything* and *Page Six*

"Vivid and poignant . . . If we as a society could only wholeheartedly embrace Dr. Sederer's sage recommendations to shift our resources from interdiction and punishment to scientifically informed prevention and treatment, we could undoubtedly escape the grip of our current opioid epidemic, mitigate the harms from other substances, and enjoy a much safer and healthier world."

—*The American Journal of Psychiatry*

"Aside from its broad insights, *The Addiction Solution* will be useful to those with afflicted loved ones."

—*The Wall Street Journal*

"Just what I needed to understand more about the opioid crisis."

—*Well + Good*

"*The Addiction Solution* offers guidance; it is not a textbook or exhaustive treatise. It proposes tools to fight the disease and plainly, though not overly simplistically, suggests the best means to implement them."

—*Shelf Awareness*

"Enriched with patient case studies that illustrate the complex nature of this disease, Sederer's balanced and compassionate approach makes this a valuable addition to the conversation on this timely topic."

—*Library Journal* (starred review)

"Timely and well-written . . . draws on many cultural sources to reveal the complex social and personal factors underlying addiction and encourage empathy."

—*Booklist* (starred review)

"Scholarly and informative . . . this book will prove invaluable."

—*Publishers Weekly*

"Comprehensive . . . a well-informed and accessible guide to treating addiction."

—*Kirkus Reviews*

THE
ADDICTION
SOLUTION

**TREATING OUR DEPENDENCE
ON OPIOIDS AND OTHER DRUGS**

LLOYD I. SEDERER, MD

SCRIBNER
New York London Toronto Sydney New Delhi

Scribner
An Imprint of Simon & Schuster, Inc.
1230 Avenue of the Americas
New York, NY 10020

First Scribner trade paperback edition February 2019

SCRIBNER and design are registered trademarks of The Gale Group, Inc., used
under license by Simon & Schuster, Inc., the publisher of this work.

For information about special discounts for bulk purchases, please contact Simon &
Schuster Special Sales at 1-866-506-1949 or business@simonandschuster.com.

The Simon & Schuster Speakers Bureau can bring authors to your live event. For
more information or to book an event, contact the Simon & Schuster Speakers
Bureau at 1-866-248-3049 or visit our website at www.simonspeakers.com.

Interior design by Jill Putorti

Manufactured in the United States of America

10 9 8 7 6 5 4 3 2 1

The Library of Congress has cataloged the hardcover edition as follows:

Names: Sederer, Lloyd I., author.
Title: The addiction solution : treating our dependence on opioids and other drugs / by
Lloyd I. Sederer, MD.
Description: First Scribner hardcover edition. | New York : Scribner, 2018. |
    Includes bibliographical references and index.
Identifiers: LCCN 2017061754| ISBN 9781501179440 (hc) | ISBN 9781501179457 (tp) |
ISBN 9781501179464 (ebook)
Subjects: LCSH: Drug abuse—Treatment—Popular works. | Substance abuse—Treatment—
Popular works. | Opioid abuse—Treatment—Popular works.
Classification: LCC RC564.29 .S43 2018 | DDC 362.29—dc23
LC record available at https://lccn.loc.gov/2017061754

ISBN 978-1-5011-7944-0
ISBN 978-1-5011-7945-7 (pbk)
ISBN 978-1-5011-7946-4 (ebook)

Photograph and diagram credits: p. 46, Photograph No. 1667921; "President Richard Nixon
Shaking Hands with Elvis Presley in the Oval Office," December 1970; Nixon White House
Photographs, 1/20/1969–8/9/1974; White House Photo Office Collection (Nixon Administra-
tion), 1/20/1969–8/9/1974; National Archives Catalog; p. 61, National Institute on Drug Abuse,
National Institutes of Health, U.S. Department of Health and Human Services; p. 88, courtesy of
the National Neuroscience Curriculum Initiative (http://www.NNCIonline.org); p. 106, the Kaiser
Family Foundation (http://www.kff.org/disparities-policy/issue-brief/beyond-health-care-the-role
-of-social-determinants-in-promoting-health-and-health-equity), Creative Commons Attribution—
NonCommercial—NoDerivatives 4.0 International License; p. 152, joshya/Shutterstock.com

To all those doing the hard work of making recovery possible—individuals, families, friends, clinicians, and policy makers

CONTENTS

AUTHOR'S NOTE

In 1955, the great director Otto Preminger released a timeless film about addiction. *The Man with the Golden Arm* took us into the life of a card dealer and aspiring drummer hooked on heroin and trying to get clean. This three-time Oscar-nominated film starred Frank Sinatra, Kim Novak, and other well-known period actors; the score, by Elmer Bernstein, was a concert unto itself.

With cinema verité, truth in film, Preminger boldly conveys the dark days of a man released from prison and determined not to go back to injecting his "golden arm" with his most powerful source of comfort. First he fails, drawn to old haunts and toxic characters, and subject to disappointments and his own deeply ingrained habits. Then, with the help of a woman, he struggles to put the demon drug, the "monkey on this back," once again behind him.

The Man with the Golden Arm is as current today as it was over sixty years ago. We witness, through this film, the power of a substance—in this instance a natural opioid, heroin—to pirate away a life, the waste in using the correctional system as a "solution," the hard work of recovery, and the inestimable value of love and support in rebuilding a life.

America is a country with a golden arm.

The regular uses of psychoactive drugs have reached their highest levels ever in the United States over this past decade.

AUTHOR'S NOTE

The use and abuse of drugs, drugs that act on our cerebral nerve cells and neural circuits, our brains and our minds, extends from the legal to the illegal purchase and distribution of substances. The biggest culprits include prescription opioid pain pills; natural and synthetic opioids such as heroin, morphine, and now fentanyl; stimulants, including Adderall, Ritalin, cocaine, and crystal meth; marijuana and its toxic synthetic relatives such as K2 or spice; ecstasy; ketamine; and many others. To avoid a boundless scope of discussion, I will mostly confine my discussion to illegal drugs and the abuse of legal drugs, particularly opioid pain pills, even though tobacco and alcohol are among the most deadly of all intoxicants.

The evidence for the escalating dominance of opioids is in their sales figures and the deaths they have induced.

Sales of prescription opioids in the United States were four times greater in 2010 than they were in 1999, and overdose deaths in 2008 were four times their rate twenty years earlier. The greatest increases in recent years have been first in the American Midwest, then in the Northeast and South, and especially among non-Hispanic whites and among those twenty-six years of age and older. Drug overdose deaths today exceed motor vehicle accidents and gunshot wounds as preventable causes of mortality, with 52,404 lethal drug overdoses identified in 2015—and this is likely an underestimate. Over 60 percent of these avoidable deaths are related to prescription pain pills and their common progression of use, abuse, and dependency, namely snorting or shooting up available, cheaper, and more potent heroin and lately the more deadly synthetic opioid fentanyl. (Overdose deaths from this and related opioids tripled from 3,105 in 2013 to 9,580 in 2015, also likely underestimates.)

The Centers for Disease Control (CDC) has declared opioids an "epidemic," as it has with more familiar epidemics such as tuberculosis, flu, and Ebola. Epidemics mean a lot of people get sick and die. We have crossed the Rubicon in America into uncharted and perilous territory.

On the legal-drug economic front, Cardinal Health allegedly shipped 241 million opioid pills to West Virginia alone from 2007 to 2012. The rates of costly hospital admissions for a substance use disorder in 2009 were six times what they were in 1999. Estimates are that four out of five first-time users of heroin first abused prescription opioids, prescribed and recreationally, only to discover they could no longer financially support their pill habit and that heroin was the "answer" to their cravings and the discomfort of withdrawal. In 2012 alone, 259 million opioid prescriptions were written—a supply that could medicate all the adults in the United States. We have never before seen this state of affairs.

The illegal-drug business today makes the Mafia's operations during Prohibition, when they made their early fortunes and established their ongoing notoriety, look like small change. The world economies nowadays annually spend an estimated $100 billion to combat the drug cartels, $20 billion federally in the United States, with methods such as crop eradication and border interdiction, yet the actual impact on costs for the cartels and the overall supply of drugs for users has over time been in the range of zero. This wasted money does not include the massive criminal justice costs for nonviolent drug offenses that the United States has expended for decades, targeting particularly people of color and those living in poverty. The costs from drug use and abuse—from family disruption, domestic violence, lost productivity (and lost taxable income), and short- and long-term disability—are legion and probably incalculable.

Complex problems, as is the addiction epidemic seizing this country, do not bend to simple or singular solutions, nor trying to police our way out of health and social problems. We need a new mind-set, one that recognizes that drugs serve a purpose, often very well, if only transiently. We need and can achieve solutions that include the person with the problem, the nature of substances themselves, and an approach informed by public health that has successfully served the world through many an epidemic. Those are what I will provide in this book.

My aim is not to alarm you, but to get your attention. We have a huge, unprecedented complex of problems regarding psychoactive drugs, especially opioids, which calls for the use of effective prevention, early intervention, and treatment initiatives to save our families, friends, and communities. We must stop doing what does not work and do more of what does. That is why I wrote this book.

INTRODUCTION

Substance use, abuse, and dependence are like a plague in this country and throughout the world. We are losing not just our children to this disease, but brothers, sisters, parents, friends, coworkers, and neighbors. The body count from overdose deaths and of productive, rewarding lives lost to addiction continues to rise. We have yet to implement solutions that will deliver what is needed to overcome the addictive forces that are eroding our societies.

A major reason why we are failing is a dogged attachment to ideas and efforts that have not worked in beating the plague of addiction. Addiction is still here, unabated. The money we are paying—in this country and throughout the globe—is not just vast; it has sadly often been wasted on unsuccessful campaigns of drug control and on education efforts that rely on stressing the negative consequences of drug use.

I believe that the biggest problem with so many of the psychoactive drugs, those that work on our brains and minds, is that they are so effective. In immediate and powerful ways they change how we feel, how we think, and how we relate and behave. That's why we use them, why "just saying no" to them is naïve and ineffective, and why the dilemma of drug taking, legal and illicit, has become one of the most dominant societal problems we face in the twenty-first century.

1

The appreciation that drugs serve a human purpose, and that we are all human, is fundamental to ending the drug epidemic we are in. This perspective, as commonsensical as it may appear, has not informed drug policy and practice in this country. When it gains traction, so shall we—and that will save many lives and countless dollars.

Take psychostimulants, for example. Countless well-designed studies on the effects of drugs such as Ritalin, Adderall, and Dexedrine on youth with hyperactive and attentional problems have shown their robust effects. Kids quiet down, can focus, and become less disruptive in classrooms within an hour of taking a psychostimulant. The use of Ritalin and Adderall is pervasive in colleges and universities; ask any student, who will tell you the truth. These drugs, in the short term, increase focus and attention and awaken sleepy brains. Youth, parents, teachers, and doctors may debate the pros and cons of their use, but are, nevertheless, left to confront the reality of a given child's or young adult's need for something that can enhance the capacity to learn and behave.

Opioids, as another example, have both legal and illegal applications as pain medications and street drugs. Among the most popular are OxyContin, Percodan, Vicodin, morphine, heroin, and now fentanyl as well. Opium has been the old standard, used in Asia for a long time but less common in the United States. We have a CDC-recognized epidemic of addiction to prescription opioids, with its consequent deadly overdoses, which has recently been joined by the recurrence of heroin use and mixed street concoctions that are even more lethal. The casualties are no longer solely the inner-city poor and people of color, but extend to white people, the middle class, and Middle America.

We need to comprehend and appreciate how these substances serve the user: that the warm opioid rush rivals any other state of euphoria and dissolves psychic and physical pain. That stimulants boost energy, focus, and mood among youth and adults. That marijuana acts as an anxiolytic, "lysing" nervousness. That alcohol is the universal solvent to unglue social inhibitions.

In my career as a psychiatrist I have cared for and overseen the treatment of tens of thousands of patients suffering from the ravages of addiction. All used drugs for perfectly intelligible reasons—because the substance served their particular needs.

I cannot think of a time in the over forty years I have been practicing psychiatry when I did not encounter, usually daily, drug use, abuse, and dependence in the patients I cared for, either directly as their doctor, as a clinical-service or hospital director, or today as a public-health official.

Drug use can appear as a primary condition in people, say alcoholism, or dependence on opioids or tranquilizers, or the compulsive use of cocaine or crystal meth. In these people, from persistent use a substance has gained control of their neurobiology and psychology. Compulsive behaviors, such as video gaming, gambling, and sex, can have the same power over our brains. Approaches to helping these people will be discussed throughout this book.

More often, because of my professional concentration on people with primary mental disorders, I have also seen the use of substances by substantial numbers of patients with what we call a co-occurring condition, also termed a comorbidity. Some experts consider the use of substances by people with serious mental illnesses to be a form of "self-medication," a way of chemically treating the anxiety, despair, difficulties concentrating and thinking, and other symptoms they experience. I find that often, but not always, to be the case, but that is more an academic than a clinical matter. We know that both the mental and the substance use disorders must be clinically detected and properly diagnosed, and that the patient must be engaged in a comprehensive treatment for both conditions. A focus on only one means the patient will not recover from either.

At the end of this book I tell the story of one of my early-career and deepest experiences with a man with the substance use disorder of alcoholism. That seared into my mind the power of psychoactive substances. When a resident, I saw how drug use was ubiquitous among the Vietnam veterans I worked with at a VA hospital, as both a primary condition and co-occurring disorder. When I moved to Boston to head up the inpatient psychiatry service at the Massachusetts General Hospital, many of our patients were reliant on alcohol and pills to bear their physical and psychic pain. Subsequently, in Cambridge, Massachusetts, where I worked with diverse populations at both Cambridge and Mount Auburn Hospitals, we were always on the lookout for the use of alcohol, marijuana, tranquilizers, and heroin, not only in the homeless but also in Boston and Cambridge undergraduates and their professors.

I then went on to be the medical director of McLean Hospital, a Harvard teaching hospital in a town adjacent to Cambridge, renowned for its services and its care of VIPs. My job was not only to see that Harvard, MIT, and the myriad other Boston schools had a place to turn when one of their students or faculty became suicidal, psychotic, or went into alcohol or drug withdrawal. I also was able to open the hospital to patients living in poverty and on entitlements, because mental and substance use disorders don't select only the rich; everyone is vulnerable. At McLean we ran a good-size clinical and research program for the treatment and study of addictions, including inpatient, residential, and outpatient services. And the many other mental health programs at McLean became skilled at identifying and treating co-occurring substance use conditions, in which a patient often used multiple drugs, though the patient would tend to prefer one drug if given the choice (often called the drug of choice).

My professional work then became principally in public health, first as the New York City mental health commissioner for five years, and now for over ten years as chief medical officer of the New York State Office of Mental Health, the largest state mental health agency in the country. One of my signature programs as New York City commissioner was to introduce buprenorphine (Suboxone) to primary-care and mental health/addiction services throughout the city. Buprenorphine had just been federally approved and represented the first novel treatment for heroin (and opioid) addiction since the early 1960s. It was safer than methadone, and likely more acceptable to people with opioid addiction because they would not need to go to a clinic daily and be observed swallowing their dose of medication. I became immersed in the world of addiction in its epicenter of New York City.

As the New York State chief mental health medical officer, from the start I worked with the state sister agency that specializes in addictions, the New York State Office of Alcoholism and Substance Abuse Services (OASAS). Our goal has been that all our respective clinics would screen for a co-occurring mental or addiction problem and ensure that our patients would be offered treatment for both, if at all possible in one setting. In recent years, with the opioid epidemic raging, I have worked with a number of state agencies and community services to enable New York to respond effectively and promptly to this deadly problem. Our work continues.

I also see in some of my family members, friends, and colleagues problems with substances—in people of all ages, including seniors. That is because the use and abuse of drugs is all around us. It now knows no socioeconomic, racial, or ethnic boundaries. That means if we look closely, we all will see these problems in people we love, befriend, and work with. I know that my work ahead will call for even more attention, in policy and programs, aimed at helping New Yorkers, all Americans, to not get caught in the epidemic of addiction and to avoid the profound suffering and personal and familial ravages it brings. I believe that addiction has become one of the major social issues of this century. That drives my work and my writing.

Drug abuse and addiction need to be recognized as a perennial human problem. Through my work, I have come to understand that a complicated mixture of social forces and biological predispositions makes some people more susceptible than others to drug abuse and addiction, and understanding those factors is the first step in prevention and treatment. (We'll go deeper into this subject in chapters 1 and 2.) We have reached an apogee in drug use, quantifiable in both deaths and dollars, but the disease of addiction is not a recent development: Americans have had a considerable appetite for drugs and alcohol since the European landings in the New World and the founding fathers. Drug use was common among Native Americans in religious ceremonies and in rites of passage, and alcohol was pervasive in Britain, quickly spreading to the New World. Furthermore, opioids—including derivatives of the poppy such as opium and morphine—have been available since the beginning of the nineteenth century, when laudanum and "black drop" opium were available by prescription and contained in many patent medicines. Heroin and the synthetic opioids have become our current scourge.

Attitudes about opioid use shifted over the nineteenth and twentieth centuries from medical acceptance to moral and legal condemnation. Nevertheless, use has remained constant.

Our railroads were built by Chinese immigrants dependent on opium, ingesting it to sustain their stamina, abate their physical pains, and quiet the sufferings of displacement. (Today, we have countless middle-aged, high school–educated, unemployed white men, many who worked with their bodies in construction and heavy-labor jobs, who use narcotic pain pills and are dying from the opioid epidemic in cities and countrysides throughout the United States.) Epidemics of the abuse of heroin, invented by Bayer in 1898, were declared after World Wars I and II and the Vietnam War. In the decades after World War II, heroin was the principal opioid drug of abuse in this country—but no longer.

The real news is the extraordinary rise in prescriptions of opioid pain pills, and with that, the explosion of use, abuse, and dependence on them that has swept this country. Deaths from overdoses of opioid prescription medications have far exceeded those of heroin for over fifteen years, though heroin overdoses have escalated considerably in recent years.

Today, we no longer have the contained problems of opioid (and other) substance use that characterized our country for two hundred years. By 2013, opioid sales and dependence had exceeded dependence on either alcohol, cocaine, and marijuana. Deaths from opioids have now exceeded those from motor vehicle accidents and gunshot wounds, combined. This isn't the tide coming in: it's a tsunami.

The dilemma of what to do about the pervasive use of substances that so effectively deliver their chemical and psychological effects, explaining their popularity, extends to alcohol, tobacco, hallucinogens, and a diverse group of prescription and illicit psychoactive drugs. This dilemma has been heightened by what has clearly been the failure of drug-control, interdiction, and criminalization policies—which disproportionately and negatively impact the poor and people of color. I am not calling for either blanket legalization of drugs or for criminalizing nonviolent users. We must, instead, reach a better understanding of how to better allocate the precious resources currently being expended. There is no significant—and certainly not sufficient—new money for prevention and treatment programs. Where will the resources come from for these critically needed actions if not from the waste resulting from ineffective strategies of drug control?

Efforts to prevent use and scare users into abstinence by stressing the negative consequences of drug use have also failed, and examination of these failed policies and practices has yet to result in substantive change. We remain too sadly stuck in puritanical, punitive, and ideological approaches to drug use, and our policies have followed. For all the human and social damages opioids and other drugs have wrought, no substantive relief seems in sight—especially if this country continues to pursue politically driven solutions rather than those drawn from science and public-health practices.

This book starts with the premise that people use drugs for good reasons: because of their desired—their needed—effects. The behavior of the users serves a purpose; however limited it may be, it is the best they know of so far. That understanding must be our starting point for changing individual drug use and abuse, prescribing practices, family and social attitudes, and governmental policies. Let's embark on that trip together. Let's recognize and follow the policy and practice innovations that will take addiction far away from our towns and families.

PS: Please note that the names and identities of all people I have cared for that are discussed in this book are fictional and meant to protect their privacy.

PART ONE

WHAT COUNTS

TEN THINGS THAT MATTER

That humanity at large will ever be able to dispense with Artificial Paradises seems very unlikely. Most men and women lead lives at the worst so painful, at the best so monotonous, poor and limited that the urge to escape, the longing to transcend themselves if only for a few moments, is and has always been one of the principal appetites of the soul. Art and religion, carnivals and saturnalia, dancing and listening to oratory—all these have served, in H. G. Wells's phrase, as Doors in the Wall.

—ALDOUS HUXLEY, *THE DOORS OF PERCEPTION*

. . . to understand how and why certain users had lost control I would have to tackle the all-important question of how and why so many others had managed to achieve control and maintain it.

—NORMAN ZINBERG, *DRUG, SET, AND SETTING*

One unpleasant consideration for those whose drug views and policies call for total abstinence is the substantial number of individuals who use but do not abuse psychoactive substances. These include people who drink alcohol in modest amounts as well as those who periodically use opioids.

Over time, as more people who take drugs own up to their use, we have reliable information about "chippers," occasional users of opioids, as well as those who use other drugs periodically without damaging their bodies, their relationships, their work, and their lives. This finding extends to occasional users of psychedelic drugs such as psilocybin, ayahuasca, peyote, and LSD.

We are still learning about marijuana as it has become legalized for recreational use by adults in eight US states and the District of Columbia, and decriminalized extensively. But the same cannot be said for tobacco or for persistent, heavy drinking, both of which cause damage to vital organs.

General statements belie the nuances and variation of response to psychoactive agents within a population of individuals. We are still left to try to understand adequately the critical dimensions of a person's biology, psychology, and community that shape any given individual's actual drug experience and use over time.

One remarkable story comes to mind. William Stewart Halsted, MD (1852–1922), was an American surgeon who was one of the four founders of Johns Hopkins Hospital. He became its first chief of surgery when it opened in 1889. Born of privilege and Ivy League educated, he was an early champion of proper aseptic techniques and the use of anesthesia for surgical procedures. He pioneered the introduction of radical mastectomies for breast cancer. Halsted performed one of the first successful gallbladder operations in the United States—in the middle of the night on his mother on her kitchen table—and delivered one of the first blood transfusions. (He transfused his own blood to his sister whom he then operated on, saving her life.) He initiated surgical training internships and residencies, which fortunately continue to this day. These are only a handful of his contributions to modern medicine. Yet throughout his distinguished medical career, Dr. Halsted was a daily drug user. First it was cocaine, an available legal local anesthetic; his "addiction" to it was treated at a Rhode Island asylum. There he was given morphine, also legal in his time, as an alternative drug, which then became his lifelong chemical partner. He injected morphine daily, all the while performing surgery and leading an exceptionally gifted and energetic life. He had some problems— would, for instance, apparently go missing from time to time— but evidently did not appreciably suffer the ravages of an opioid addiction nor a serious, deleterious effect on his health, family, or achievements.

I clearly am not advocating a morphine habit as the path to a famed life. Instead, Halsted's example, along with many others, compels us to look beyond the pharmacology of any given drug to understand how it may or may not affect the life of the person who uses it.

Below I identify ten factors that influence how an individual will interact with a psychoactive substance. My purpose is to try to fill in the information gaps and correct some of the misinformation that clouds our thinking about substances. My goal is to more intelligently inform how we feel about, respond to, and set social policy for those who use drugs as well as their families, friends, and communities.

I address these ten, which are not of equal valence, in a limited fashion and not in order of importance. While there are other factors, these are salient.

1. AGE

The human brain does not complete its maturation until well into the third decade of life, later for males than for females. Appreciating the protracted development of the human brain can help parents understand the emotional volatility, impulsivity, and potential for poor judgment that drives youth, especially adolescents. It also is a caution about the use of substances while the brain is developing, laying down the myelin that braces our nerve fibers and helps us make better decisions.

The regular use of marijuana in teenage years may indeed impair intellectual, academic, and athletic performance. In addition, in youth with a biological predisposition to psychotic illness, its use can unleash an underlying mental disorder. The use of drugs, alcohol, and cigarettes in adolescence can also signal a greater propensity for their use in later years. Teens who smoke cigarettes by the time they are eighteen are far more likely to use tobacco when they're older. (Smoking remains the greatest preventable cause of morbidity and mortality in developed countries.)

There are similar considerations for alcohol use, which is pervasive among American teenagers despite being illegal. Its limited use, without bingeing or overdose, usually turns into the social-drinking patterns that characterize most adults. Genetic traits and experiences of alcohol, positive and negative in a family, can tip the balance and foster dependence on this substance—or not—as a youth matures. Early drinking is a marker of biological vulnerability to alcohol as well as to individual and family social malaise. Preventing use in vulnerable teens as well as early detection of and intervention for problem drinking and drug taking are age-specific actions that can make a lifetime of difference.

2. SET

Billie Holiday (1915–59) was arguably one of the greatest blues singers. I happen to think so. Johann Hari, in his remarkable and bestselling book *Chasing the Scream*, eloquently tells her story, which I summarize here. When Billie was born, her mother was nineteen and her father seventeen, but he was nowhere to be found. Billie's mother was a prostitute, and the streets of Baltimore became Billie's home from an early age. When ten, she was raped. Her screams brought the police, who concluded she was also a prostitute. (Imagine alleging a ten-year-old to be prostituting herself?) She was briefly jailed and soon mandated to a year in a reform school. While there, as punishment for her lack of obedience, she was locked in an empty room overnight with a dead body; no one answered her screams. She escaped and fled to Harlem, in New York City, where she thought her mother might have gone. Indeed, her mother was working in a brothel, would not keep her, and threw her out. Billie's "solution," as a fourteen-year-old, was to prostitute herself, first in a brothel and then for a violent pimp whom her mother urged her to marry.

It gets worse. She was arrested for prostitution and sent to prison on Welfare Island, now Roosevelt Island, the predecessor institution to Rikers Island. When she was released, her first objective was to ingest the most powerful substances she could find, first high-proof, cheap alcohol, and soon heroin. Her habit would transport her away from a mind filled with rape, imprisonment, physical violence, and maternal neglect. She looked for work, failed as a dancer, but, boy, could she carry a tune. Billie the singer was born.

But she continued under the "management" of her abusive pimp (and husband), who stole her money and reportedly punched her in the face after one of her storied performances at Carnegie Hall. She continued to drink heavily and shoot heroin. She became the special target of one Harry Anslinger—whose story is bracingly told by Alexandra Chasin in *Assassin of Youth*—the first director of the Federal Bureau of Narcotics, the successor agency to the former Department of Prohibition, which had no Prohibition left to enforce.

Billie was set up to be busted by her pimp-husband, who wanted her punished. She was sent to prison again, this time in West Virginia, for a year. As a consequence of her crime she lost her cabaret license and became homeless—though her legend continued. She found gigs outside of standard clubs until she once again was pursued by the Feds and arrested in San Francisco in what appears to have been a drug plant by federal agents, who entered her room without a search warrant. She was acquitted at trial, but her life spiraled further down. She had cirrhosis of the liver from the alcoholism and remained addicted to heroin. She died in a hospital at the age of forty-four, afraid that the Feds would send her to prison again, to make her an example of the perils of drug addiction.

Imagine the first moments that this heavenly songstress—raped, beaten, abandoned, neglected, imprisoned, and without prospects—knocked down her first strong drink or felt the warmth and comfort of heroin coursing through her veins. It is a bit of a miracle that some escape a life like hers without alcohol or drug dependence—but too many, like Billie, don't. Her psychic pain became the driver of her addiction, the ingredient that made her encounter with psychoactive drugs necessary and irresistible.

Set means a personal vulnerability to drugs, which has two components: first, personality, the preexisting character of a person, fashioned by their life story and including any tendency to externalize or hold circumstances and other people responsible for any problems; and second, an individual's unique biological responsiveness to any given drug.

In work supported by the National Institute on Drug Abuse (NIDA) in the 1970s, when this concept was postulated and popularized, set was more specifically defined for research purposes.

Five personality dimensions were studied: passive vs. active; intimacy vs. isolation; rebelliousness vs. conformity; awareness of affect vs. distance from affect (feelings); and distortion of reality vs. its acceptance. Moreover, attention focused on the indicia of early personality problems such as delinquent and criminal behavior as well as troubled family backgrounds. This research revealed the qualities of people that can shape the set of their use and their experience when taking drugs. The person who takes the drug is an active "ingredient" in his or her response, for immediate as well as longer-term effects.

In the late sixties and in the seventies, inspired by a culture of "turn on and tune out," the ingestion of LSD (as well as other drugs) became popular. For a number of years urban emergency departments (EDs) were populated by young people in the throes of a "bad trip." A scare spread about the danger of LSD, and its potential to destroy the minds of its users. But then, a few years later, EDs would rarely see a bad trip. What happened? It was not the drug, it was the psychological state that people using had been in upon ingesting the LSD. Their fear and misinformation, their psychological set, produced the panic that infused their drug experience. Over time, LSD subcultures educated users about how to use it, how not to panic, and to take the drug in environments conducive to calm and security, with guides to help smooth out the bumps. The set had been altered—and the drug experience went from what had been a nightmare to a pleasant reverie.

I do not mean to suggest that anyone who is well prepared for the use of a psychedelic drug and takes LSD in a sweet setting with good and experienced drug-using friends can ingest it with impunity. Some people with latent or preexisting serious mental disorders, including schizophrenia and bipolar disorder, are at high risk of unleashing a psychotic state that may persist well after LSD has left their body. This exemplifies a *biological* set or disposition, different from a *psychological* set, where the mental state of the user will powerfully influence what happens when a drug is ingested.

3. SETTING

In 1971, Dr. Norman Zinberg, of Cambridge Hospital and Harvard Medical School, was asked by the Department of Defense and the Ford Foundation to go to Vietnam, where a deeply unpopular and deadly war was raging. He was an expert on drugs, whose work I greatly admired when I worked in the same psychiatry department, and his mission was to assess the degree to which combat soldiers were using heroin and advise on what might be done. A worry was that when the soldiers came home, they would bring their habits with them, outnumbering the estimated total of those already addicted to heroin in the United States.

From reports by Zinberg and his collaborator Lee Robins, about 20 percent of the enlisted men in Vietnam were using heroin frequently, from daily to many times a week. They had access to potent, uncontaminated, cheap heroin, which they principally smoked or snorted. This psychiatrist and psychiatric epidemiologist, working together, forecast that the soldiers' drug use would be largely left behind in the jungles of Southeast Asia after they came back to the United States. And they were right. Eighty-eight percent of the returning soldiers who used did not continue to do so. Though 12 percent did, in excess of the rates of the general population, these men had battled in a guerrilla, tropical war that lacked support at home and from the people they were ostensibly trying to "save." Many were seeking a means to "make time go away." Moreover, we know today that up to 30 percent of battle-exposed veterans develop PTSD, clinical depression, traumatic brain injury (TBI), or all three—coupled with high rates of alcohol and drug use related to these conditions.

All this is what is meant by setting, in which the context, the environment, and the circumstances are fundamental to a person's use, abuse, and dependence on a drug. We are in the dark unless we shine a light on the setting in which a psychoactive drug is employed.

4. ROUTE OF ADMINISTRATION

The faster a substance gets into our brain, the more likely it is to become habit-forming.

The tobacco in cigarettes has perhaps the most rapid form of administration of any substance, which helps make cigarettes among the most addictive of substances and the hardest to quit. Much the same can be said of crystal meth and cocaine when they are smoked, the latter as crack cocaine. Some experts and drug users remark that it is easier to quit heroin than cigarettes, and a 2010 scientific report to the EU declared tobacco to have a substantially greater risk of causing addiction than heroin, alcohol, cocaine, or cannabis. Yet Alcoholics and Narcotics Anonymous (AA and NA) seem to accept addiction to tobacco as an exception to their prominent aim of achieving abstinence.

Cocaine snorted is less addictive than cocaine rolled into a cigarette and smoked. When cocaine is crystallized and smoked as crack, potent amounts even more rapidly reach the brain, where they have a short but intense effect that fosters repeated use and dependence. Methamphetamine is a common, available stimulant that has been used recreationally and to improve academic performance, and to a lesser extent as a treatment for attention deficit/hyperactivity disorder. But its illegal crystallized form, crystal methamphetamine (meth), evokes incredible energy and euphoria that is so rewarding, especially when the drug is inhaled, that the user often repeatedly chases the (initial) high. But that first-time nirvana is seldom reachieved, while the repetitive use of the drug can be destructive, toxic to our brain cells. This drug was popularized in the hugely successful TV show *Breaking Bad*.

Our brains seem to become more habituated to substances that arrive immediately, powerfully, and that don't last long. The route of administration counts when it comes to how we humans respond to substances.

5. PURITY

The critical issue is not really purity but *impurity*. Pharmaceutical morphine, the kind that Dr. Halsted used, lacked contaminants and was not laced with other substances such as talcum powder, strychnine, or fentanyl. As a result, he was not poisoned by the impurities that are almost always found in illicit drugs, especially those sold down the drug distribution chain.

Harm-reduction approaches to drug addiction seek to provide users with safer forms of the drug, lacking in potential poisons, as well as with clean needles. The reductions in the transmission of HIV and hepatitis C, as well as in overdoses and toxic reactions, which can be fatal, from harm-reduction programs are impressive.

6. POTENCY

The concept is straightforward and the salience great. Our brains are physiologically organized to react through the neurotransmitters and neural circuits that chemically and electrically drive mental operations, including how we feel and think. The stronger the stimulus, in the form of a powerful exogenous substance, the bigger the neural bang.

Substances such as cocaine, nicotine, and methamphetamine stimulate dopamine release, especially in the nucleus accumbens (NAc), a region in each hemisphere of the brain that has a role in feelings of aversion, pleasure, reward, and certain forms of learning associated with drug seeking. All addictive substances produce dopamine release in the NAc, presumably because the receptors they directly target (cannabinoid, opioid, nicotinic, etc.) are all connected to the brain reward system. The dopamine release produces the pleasurable high that characterizes the drug experience, at least early on.

Ingested opioids act on μ-opioid (pronounced *mu*) receptors in the brain and intestinal tract and can reduce pain and produce euphoria and narcosis (sedation), as well as cause reduced libido and constipation.

Cannabinoid receptors are more widely located and exist throughout the body and brain. They are instrumental to mood, memory, pain, and appetite. Marijuana specifically targets these receptors. Marijuana began its ascent to popularity with musicians and artists well before the 1960s, when the youth culture of the Western world discovered its sweet effects on our mood and its capacity to open many a door of perception. Now eight US states and the District of Columbia have legalized its recreational use, and more than half the states have some form of legal medicinal marijuana. Huge policy issues face this country (and other nation-states) on whether to decriminalize or legalize; on how to grow and ensure quality control for safety and dose; on what regulations, taxes, and distribution channels are needed and at what cost; and more.

Drugs such as marijuana, which are used by so many (and greater access will likely increase their use), may have medicinal utility and can produce fewer problems than alcohol or opioids, but they too have negative consequences, especially for the developing brain of adolescents (and fetuses in utero) and when used in high doses over long periods. In the years ahead we will need to observe and record carefully how greater access to cannabis may affect its use and abuse, and what ill health it may deliver. We have, in effect, a national, natural experiment about marijuana going on in the United States. If we systematically study it, with science not ideology, we will be able to enlighten future policy decisions about this drug.

Whatever the drug, its effects are often linearly correlated with the amount taken—which means that a person's response is in part determined by taking more or using a more potent concoction, or both. Think of "proof" for alcoholic beverages, a measure of the percentage of ethanol in a type of alcoholic beverage: 80-proof vodka, for example, has 40 percent alcohol; beers typically have 3–10 percent, and wines 4–13 percent. A person has to drink far less vodka than beer to raise his or her blood alcohol level and get the brain intoxicated. Fentanyl, a commonly used, legal opioid anesthetic, is fifty to a hundred times more powerful than morphine—which explains why it is so often present in the blood of people who die of accidental drug overdoses. They never knew what hit them.

Ingesting high doses of a drug, another way of increasing its potency in the body, can produce toxic psychotic states. We see this with cocaine, hashish, belladonna, and even alcohol.

Potency matters, whatever the agent. Higher potency can enhance the desired response as well as amplify unintended consequences, which range from bothersome constipation to the cessation of breathing.

7. HALF-LIFE

Alprazolam, or Xanax, was introduced in the United States in 1969. A benzodiazepine, a class of drugs that includes Librium, Valium, and Klonopin, Xanax quickly became among the five bestselling drugs in the United States and has done well since then. It has sometimes been called vitamin X.

I recall prescribing Xanax for patients with significant anxiety and for people with severe depression until they experienced some symptomatic relief from treatment with antidepressants and therapy; with some other patients I used Xanax to help them with their fear of flying. But I assiduously avoided giving it to people with substance-abuse problems because, as a "benzo," it could be habit-forming.

The half-life of a drug is defined as the time required for the body's blood levels of the substance to decrease by half. For Xanax, reportedly it is about eleven hours on average, in a range that goes from six to twenty-seven hours, reflecting how different individuals metabolize the drug. Clinically, many patients seem to feel its waning effects toward the lower end of the time range.

Many patients I treated would report Xanax "wearing off" in just a few hours and then their feeling even more anxious. They wanted to know if they could take more sooner. They were experiencing withdrawal from the drug, not likely the breakthrough of their underlying psychiatric disorder. Patients found it exceedingly hard to stop using Xanax, even after a few weeks; the dose kept having to be halved, with even the lowest-dose pills broken into tiny particles, before patients could finally quit. This problem with Xanax, which many but not all experience, is now well-known and has led many doctors to prefer benzos with far longer half-lives (such as Klonopin, or clonazepam as a generic).

Behavioral views of addiction importantly stress *both* its negative and positive aspects. Negative reinforcement is seen when drug levels decrease in the body, which can be terminated by taking the drug. Positive reinforcement refers to effects on the brain's reward system, including releasing dopamine and other neurotransmitters. Anyone, but especially someone with an addiction, will seek the reward (e.g., euphoria) or to avoid the pain (reductions in blood levels and withdrawal).

Imagine a drug with a half-life of about fifteen minutes, which is the half-life of crack cocaine, with the high maybe lasting ten minutes. The euphoria is sky-high, but the crash is intense, precipitous, and deep. The answer? Take more. Keep taking it.

Methamphetamine tablets have a half-life of about ten hours (range six to fifteen hours). When smoked as crystal meth, its "bioavailability," or capacity to be taken up by nerve and other cells, is far greater, yet this drug sticks around with a half-life similar to that of the tablets. This allows for meth "runs," in which users stay high for days on end, finally crashing into a physical and emotional abyss. The urge then, of course, is to resume using to end the agony of the crash.

For alcohol, the blood alcohol concentration (BAC) achieved from one drink decreases by 50 percent each hour, which is why our blood alcohol level keeps rising when we have a few drinks in a relatively short time. It is also why we then wake up in the middle of the night feeling the consequences of declining levels of alcohol in our bloodstream and brain, causing our nervous system to rebound from its previous state of alcohol (drug) suppression. Withdrawal is the figurative bell that awakens us in the night.

The half-life of a drug, thus, shapes our need to want more of it to achieve its benefits, and to ward off the effects of its disappearance.

8. THE PLANTS THEMSELVES

The composition of the plant from which the drug is derived also affects use and dependence. This is as true of cocaine synthesized from coca leaves as of opioids from poppies, and the timeliest example is marijuana.

Let's consider the cannabis plant. It contains scores of cannabinoids, but the two present in the highest concentrations (called phytocannabinoids) are THC (tetrahydrocannabinol) and cannabidiol.

Marijuana users seek THC to trigger the brain's naturally occurring endocannabinoid receptors, which produce the (hopefully) pleasant rush that attends this drug. But depending on the plant, a certain portion, even up to 40 percent, of the psychoactive ingredients is cannabidiol. Curiously, cannabidiol does not produce the psychological effects of its sister agent, cannabis or THC, and does not seem to significantly impair motor or cognitive performance.

Cannabidiol has been sold as a dietary supplement to control a rare form of infant-onset, intractable epilepsy (Dravet syndrome). Cannabidiol also has been reported to reduce seizures by 50 percent in some children and adults with Lennox-Gastaut syndrome, another form of severe epilepsy. Cannabidiol may also affect marijuana users' experience of the drug, even though it doesn't produce the high of THC. Some people experience psychotic reactions when using marijuana, especially people with latent or emerging schizophrenia, and higher concentrations of cannabidiol appear to help deter those reactions—and this is particularly true for those affected by schizophrenia. Studies are under way to explore if cannabidiol may be an effective antipsychotic drug, and an alternative to the common antipsychotics with their limited effectiveness and range of significant side effects.

So the plant itself can be a factor in the response we humans have to ingesting it.

9. REFINEMENT AND EXTRACTION

Dr. Andrew Weil, always a vocal proponent of natural highs, stresses refinement and extraction in his popular book *The Natural Mind*.

The coca leaf, often chewed by members of indigenous cultures for stamina, has been processed for its highly potent ingredient, cocaine. True to the adage that more means more, the effects of cocaine, especially when it reaches the brain in seconds, are greater than for coca, as are its toxic effects.

Peyote is a small cactus native to Mexico and parts of Texas. Its use by Native Americans dates back over five thousand years. Ten to twenty grams of dried peyote "buttons" (the part of the cactus that grows aboveground) can yield 200–400 mg of pure mescaline, which is the principal psychoactive substance. By drying the peyote, the more potent concoction mescaline is produced, with greater neurochemical impact. One, albeit inexact, analogy is to alcohol proof, where higher-proof alcohol blends have greater effects, desired and undesired, as does mescaline when it is used instead of the peyote plant.

Dr. Weil has much to teach us about "the natural mind" and the natural use of substances. The Paleo movement—meaning living as we humans did in the Stone Age as hunter-gatherers, in diet, exercise, not wearing shoes, and sustaining life in concert with our environment—is perhaps a good example of how far naturalistic beliefs have evolved.

I am not a proponent of only singularly prescribing substances that are "natural," but when we imbibe or consume these powerful substances, we want to know from whence they came, and how they were extracted.

10. THE DRUG/SOCIAL FORCES RATIO

We can think of this ratio as another way of looking at set and setting, when placed against the strength of the drug.

For instance, in the treatment of tobacco addiction, nicotine patches can control cravings and help a person quit, increasing the quit rate by 50–70 percent. Yet this mode of treatment appears to be effective in only 23 percent of people who try, and 15 percent after one year. Some of the limited effect of nicotine-replacement treatments may relate to their relatively short duration of use—unlike other replacement drugs that are used as maintenance, and thus for extended periods. What this nevertheless means is that more than 75 percent of the time nicotine therapy fails, illustrating that other factors, such as lack of readiness to change, limited social supports, and contact with other smokers, significantly outweigh the impact of ingesting the replacement drug.

We have seen good rates of success with methadone and buprenorphine as medication-assisted treatment for opioid addiction. But they are but one buttress against the power of environmental cues from friends, media, music, TV, and merely walking around the neighborhood, all of which can be strong triggers for drug relapse. The environment often trumps the action of a drug treatment, though medication treatment is one valuable component in a comprehensive and ongoing treatment plan for a person with an addiction.

Conversely, a safe and familiar environment with a skilled guide can result in far greater rates of good trips from LSD, psilocybin, and peyote. A good social milieu can bring out the best and safest of responses in the person ingesting these substances. The ratio of external influence to drug effect here again is on the side of the environment.

For all substances, then, we need to recognize what circumstances, what preexisting character, views, and biology, and what human supports, can outweigh a drug's noxious actions or enhance its desired effects.

My aim in this chapter has been to highlight how drugs, as powerful as they can be, may be enhanced or mitigated in their effects and altered in the user's mind and brain by a variety of personal, contextual, and neurological factors. I did not try to be comprehensive in this rendering but rather illustrative. For example, I did not discuss a number of other individual differences in humans (scientifically known as hosts), including rates of drug metabolism or how the brain changes over time with use of many of the substances discussed here.

Drug taking is a highly complex and variable human and social phenomenon. And it is not going away, prohibitionists and border interdictionists notwithstanding. Human beings throughout this planet have used psychoactive drugs since the Stone Age and, except for the Inuit until the white man came, every society has partaken—and continues to do so.

If we are to inculcate intelligence and balance in our efforts to reduce the harm or enhance the benefits of drug use, legal and illegal, one-dimensional or simplistic efforts will continue to waste time, drain personal and governmental treasuries, sustain familial and community agonies, and along the way sacrifice countless human lives.

We can tip the balance from harm to benefits—and certainly to harm reduction—from addiction to abstinence or controlled use, and from failed and destructive criminalization to decriminalization and selective legalization. But only if we open our eyes, expand our consciousness, to what really matters in the use of psychoactive substances.

2

DIMENSIONS OF CHARACTER

The good physician treats the disease; the great physician treats the patient who has the disease.

—SIR WILLIAM OSLER

Contrary to some long-held cultural beliefs, addiction is a disease—not a character weakness or a failure of will. The persistence of these prejudices may make it risky for me to discuss the dimensions of character in addiction, but as a psychiatrist I have learned that understanding people's character is a useful way of appreciating how they see the world, how they are apt to engage in relationships, how they respond when stressed, and what psychological capabilities they can bring into the work of overcoming an addiction and remaking a life of dignity and contribution. This exploration of character is another way of considering the factors that matter in addiction, here in the context of real people's psyches and lived experiences.

I recall being on call as a resident when a twenty-four-year-old man, Antonio DeLuca, was brought by ambulance to a local emergency room in the middle of the night after impulsively taking a "handful" of acetaminophen (Tylenol, which most people do not know can cause severe liver damage, even death, when consumed in excess). His sister, who had called an emergency line, said that he was famous for brief, intense attachments followed by angry disappointments with vindictive and self-destructive behaviors. His job history too was spotty and tumultuous, with a trail of angry former employers. Antonio's parents no longer welcomed him at home because he typically blamed them and was prone to steal if not watched. He episodically drank heavily and used cocaine when he could afford it.

Once medically stable, his stomach pumped and IV fluids given, he complained that his girlfriend was not taking good care of him, expected too much of him, and had ended the relationship, such as it was. He had recently, as well, lost a job as a construction worker for picking a fight with a coworker. When emergency-room professionals tried to get him to think about his next steps, he was sullen and evasive. He remarked, "If you trust anyone, they will suck you dry."

While I did not see him again after that troubling encounter, I have seen many other men and women with the same constellation of addictive and impulsive behaviors, contentious relationships with family and others, inability to sustain employment, and an externalizing view of the world, where others are always perceived to be the problem and are always responsible for any difficulties rather than the person himself. That profile does not augur well for gaining control of an addiction and making a better life, though at times I have been pleasantly surprised to see someone gain mastery, over time, and regain a proper place in the world.

I also recall, when working at Massachusetts General Hospital some time ago, a referral from a distinguished primary-care doctor of a married couple, John and Susan Noble, for consultation in my private practice. They were in their forties, and ostensibly Susan was to be the patient. She had seemed "depressed" to this referring primary-care doctor. Her husband came with her to the consultation. She was artistic, but not commercially, and ran their home and social life; he was an accomplished businessman.

At our initial meetings, Susan indeed appeared depressed and seemed from her story to have been that way for some time. She was also angry at John, who she asserted drank too heavily and was highly critical and demeaning, but not physically abusive, after a few or more cocktails, which he consumed nightly. He did not deny his alcohol use, though he tended to minimize it, and had his own complaints about his wife, which he acknowledged would surface at home when he drank. Yet he was solicitous of her and wanted to see that she got treatment for her depression.

I offered to treat Susan's depression with therapy, seeing her individually as well as periodically with her husband, given their overt dissension, as well as with an antidepressant. She politely declined, saying, "I will manage on my own," and adding that if her husband were more supportive and less disparaging, she would feel a lot better. The consultation ended there, after two ninety-minute sessions. I made it plain that my door was always open for her to return, and I let her primary-care doctor know where matters stood.

Months passed. I received a call from John. He wanted to speak with me, and I set up a time. So began a therapy with him that lasted a number of years, and an ongoing doctor-patient relationship that continued for many years thereafter, finally ending when I left Massachusetts for a position in DC. John clearly saw that he had a drinking problem, as had his deceased father. Highly educated and successful, by the time John was in his thirties his custom was to drink anywhere from several to "many" alcoholic drinks a night. By morning, he was sober and busy at his company, among the first to arrive and the last to leave. That was about all his life entailed, with some diminished socializing arranged by his wife. No close friends, no exercise, no use of his past literary talents, no pleasure in his marriage.

In the therapy, which John came to on time and ready for self-examination, he soon said he knew he needed to stop drinking. We talked about what other supports besides therapy might be useful, such as AA or disulfiram, also called Antabuse, a deterrent drug that with regular use causes a nasty reaction if alcohol is consumed. There was little else at that time, since CBT, motivational interviewing, and relapse prevention were truly in their infancy—and medications to reduce cravings had yet to be introduced.

John was concerned about his privacy and sensitive professional position and said no to AA, even though I explained that many others of his station would be in groups in downtown Boston or near his suburban home. Both of us were reluctant to use disulfiram. He said he would stop, that he could no longer face himself for how he had deteriorated and behaved—and that he wanted a better, richer life. And he did stop, completely and on a day he set in the near future.

Instead of pouring a cocktail first thing when he got home, he put on his sneakers and went for a walk, often for an hour during the week and longer on weekends. He rekindled some friendships and began writing fiction, which he loved. His marriage remained a stalemate, but he took control of what he could, namely himself and his behaviors, and it worked. He never took a drink again. Annually, he would mark the date of his sobriety for himself and let me know. For many years after I left the Boston area, he would write me to recognize another year without alcohol and to express his appreciation of our work together, and to modestly acknowledge his own achievements.

As for Susan, a couple of years after our initial consultation John said that she was ready to be treated for her depression. Since John was now my patient, I referred her to a colleague. But full remission from her depression eluded her since her ability to do the work of treatment and recovery remained limited. Medications can help, but a person typically needs to try to rebuild her life, emotionally, socially, and physically. Susan instead became more isolated and alone and developed a chronic pain syndrome that led to a dependence on opioids. John remained with her, living a parallel existence under the same roof.

We all develop enduring ways, usually well rooted by adolescence, by which we perceive, feel, think, and behave. This is what we can think of as our *character*. Character is different from the mental conditions, psychopathology, that can develop from it. In these so-called personality disorders a person's actions are persistently maladaptive and cause individual or interpersonal misery, often defying social norms. Those diagnosed with personality disorders may experience difficulties in cognition, emotions, interpersonal functioning, or impulse control. Personality disorders are diagnosed in 40–60 percent of psychiatric patients, making them the most frequent of psychiatric diagnoses.

Antonio DeLuca, described above, had the features of both borderline and paranoid personality disorders. These conditions were not serving him well in adapting to everyday life.

In understanding character in general, not its disturbances as manifested in personality disorders, psychologists have studied what is called the ego, a valuable construct in comprehending our mental operations and behavior. Early-twentieth-century analysts, especially Anna Freud (Sigmund Freud's daughter), were interested in the ego and its operations and laid down its conceptual foundations.

The ego—one component of Sigmund Freud's triad of the id, the ego, and the superego—performs a group of mental functions. When functioning well, the ego enhances everyday functioning and adaptation; when it does not, psychological symptoms and mental distress arise.

The principal functions of the ego are:

- *Reality testing*, our capacity to correctly appraise the world around us.
- *Regulating and controlling our drives*, including sex, aggression, hunger, and attachment. Limited capabilities in this function can be a big problem. We need to be able to control our drives to ensure our safety and work and social functioning. Without some good measure of collective drive control we will not be able to realize stable civilizations.
- *Maintaining human relationships*, unfortunately often still called object relations by psychoanalysts. People are not objects, and even our inner representations of others and ourselves as "objects" begs for a more humanistic term. But the role of the ego in attachment and ongoing relationships is crucial.
- *Executive mental functions*, including perception, memory, attention and concentration, sequencing and planning, abstraction and judgment. Impairment in any or many of these functions will produce disturbances in thought and behavior and erode a person's ability to lead a rewarding life.

- Last and not at all least are a set of what are called *ego defenses* or *defense mechanisms*. When these are particularly disturbed, it fosters a characteristic pattern of behaviors, known as personality disorders, including borderline and narcissistic personalities, paranoid personality, and antisocial personalities (including sociopathy).

As we consider the ego defenses carefully, we see that they cover a gradient from highly adaptive to lower levels of adaptation. Where a person sits on this continuum will reveal what we can expect of him or her, especially when stressed, as well as the person's potential to function in the world he or she lives in.

At the most highly adaptive end of the ego-defense continuum are altruism; humor; a capacity to delay; sublimation, or turning instinctual drives such as sex and aggression into virtues; affiliation with and attachment to others; and proper self-assertion. The more of these we have and can mobilize in the wake of disappointment, loss, or misfortune, the better a life we will enjoy, and the more others will enjoy us as well.

John Noble's ego generally functioned at this level, though it was prone to lose ground when intoxicated or, over time, from the mental effects of the chronic use of alcohol. He could serve others, reflect on himself, seek the support of others, delay gratification (with effort), and sublimate his self-destructive drives into physical activity and creativity.

Some people employ the defenses of isolating feelings; repression of difficult matters; excessive intellectualization; reaction formation, or doing the opposite of what we actually feel; and dissociation, which leads to numbness and a mild loss of reality testing.

Susan Noble had features of emotional isolation and had distanced herself from others. Reaction formation made her seem overly kindly when on the inside she was boiling with rage. Her perceptions of others were tinged with distrust, a mild form of compromised reality testing that left her bereft and with little hope for a better life.

Farther down the gradient are defenses that distort reality—bend it to what someone needs to believe rather than what actually is—as well as the defenses of devaluing of others and omnipotence. It is easy to see how less adaptive ego defenses can impair a life.

Even greater impaired ego functioning leads to denial and projection, holding someone else responsible for what we think and feel and for whatever trouble we are in. Psychotic states are characterized by these types of ego operations. When the ego is quite compromised, we see impulsive, destructive behaviors, passive aggression, help-rejecting complaining (*gornish helfin*, "nothing will help," in Yiddish), and emotional and interpersonal withdrawal.

At its most impaired level of functioning, the ego resorts to delusions (false, fixed ideas), psychotic denial and distortion of reality, and abandonment of a sense of agency or responsibility for the self—"It's not my fault, it's yours."

Back to Antonio. His clinical presentation showed a host of compromised ego defenses. He was impulsive, distrustful, managed feelings with substances, not sublimation, and had shattered relationships in family, love, and work. Why is it important to consider his character—not to label him with a personality disorder but to appreciate what was going on in his mind and heart? Because that is how we could engage him, join and begin to help him bend his experience of reality to what is real, and thereby enable him to start the work of treatment and recovery. I learned in psychiatry school that we need to meet people where they are and help take them where they fear to go.

It would surely have been a clinical failure to confront him about his behaviors, to stress their consequences, or to scold him. At some level he knew that and suffered with that shame. Instead, engagement—by professionals, families, and friends—starts with the premise that behavior serves a purpose. What was he achieving, the best he knew how, by his demands and contentiousness? How did these protect him, serve him? We must start here to let him, and others like him, know we appreciate his dilemma and can be there to help him rebuild his life.

With ego defenses in the psychotic range it is even more essential to not confront a person about his or her delusions or projections. Doing so will either drive that person away or evoke aggression, likely at whoever is making that mistake. Engagement starts in far more neutral ways, in understanding who people are, their sense of the world, and, over time, what they seek for themselves in life.

Drug dependence impairs ego functioning and can induce a profound defensive slide. A person can go from altruism to self-absorption, from rational, goal-directed behavior to impulsive acting out, and from capable reality testing to its opposite, namely denial and distortion. The capacity of many drugs, especially those that work on brain reward centers—such as opioids and psychostimulants—to "pirate" the brain and induce mental regression to limited, even primitive, ego states and functioning is well-known. But judge not the underlying character of a person actively in the throes of an addiction. When clean, sober, and in recovery, people can find their way back up the ego/defensive ladder and become very different. Such is the story of Dr. Robert Brown, which helps us understand the risk and protective factors that can be active in the development of an addiction.

Robert Brown, a physician, was fifty-seven when he fled his home state thinking, mistakenly, that he could elude his professional licensing board's efforts to take away his medical license.

His wife, Sandra, aided in his escape. Loyal and devoted to him, she had witnessed him change from a responsible and respected doctor to a man whose every action was aimed at obtaining opioid prescription medications for his own use. Evidence of his use emerged not just at home, but from state pharmacy data, which revealed his filling multiple prescriptions, written by different doctors throughout his state, for OxyContin and Vicodin. Dr. Brown was also using what little money the family had that wasn't already eaten away by his habit for the purchase of illicit opioids. He had not crossed the so-called needle barrier, when a substance user goes from orally taking or smoking a substance to injecting it into a vein—even though he had ready access to syringes.

The state bureau that issued his medical license first tried to persuade him to enter treatment. Many states have "impaired physician (and nurse)" programs, where doctors and nurses are identified and offered a plan in which a medical license may initially be suspended but restored when it is safe to do so. These programs, which include agreed-upon treatment, drug testing, and monitoring, are often effective, but Dr. Brown proved not yet ready and kept using. When he was told that his license would be terminated, he and his wife packed their belongings and headed to another state, imagining he could beat his addiction and start anew someplace else.

But addiction is a fierce companion and not easily shed by crossing state lines.

After the move, Dr. Brown tried to take emergency-room call to make some money and gain access to supplies of hospital opioids. But hospitals are now good at making sure a physician is properly licensed to care for patients. Unemployed and almost constantly miserable from withdrawal, Dr. Brown agreed at his wife's pleading to return to their home state and take the licensing board up on its offer to help.

Those in the field of addictions appreciate that both risk and protective factors influence whether a person will develop a substance use disorder.

Among the risk factors for addiction are a parent who relied on alcohol or drugs or had a mental illness; childhood trauma, from neglect or abuse; and adult trauma from war, forced emigration, or a natural disaster, such as a hurricane or flood. Neighborhood risk factors include poverty, unstable housing, racism, and violence. Those fortunate to have had supportive, engaged families and households free of violence and addiction benefit from these protective factors. Faith in a higher power, whether through a formal religion or not, is a strong protective factor and a vital tool in recovery for those who develop addiction and are working on their recovery. Education and employment opportunities are protective as well.

Dr. Brown grew up in a tough inner-city neighborhood. He was bullied and beaten for being a good student with aspirations. His father was an alcoholic, frequently unemployed, and given to violent outbursts at both his wife and his son when intoxicated. But as a young man Brown studied hard, was active in after-school programs, and exited his circumstances through education and faith-based activities. He had both risk and protective factors—which were instrumental in his developing a substance use disorder and his capacity to recover, respectively. Most people have a combination of both, but some, such as Billie Holiday, just have the deck stacked against them.

Opioid withdrawal is painful, though rarely life threatening—generally only so when other drugs are involved or a person has other medical illnesses that compromise cardiac or lung functioning. Dr. Brown admitted himself to a detoxification facility, where he received methadone in steadily decreasing doses to mitigate his withdrawal symptoms and thereby help keep him from going AWOL to secure drugs. In ten days he was opioid-free, and he remained for another eighteen days of a traditional twenty-eight-day program to receive counseling and attend 12-step recovery groups, Narcotics Anonymous in particular, as well as relapse prevention groups. There was a focus on healthy living as well, with attention to sleep, good nutrition, exercise, and relaxation techniques such as meditation and yoga. He did not choose medication-assisted treatment, which could probably have been buprenorphine, which attaches to the brain's opioid receptors and helps to control cravings.

On discharge from the detox program, Dr. Brown continued counseling, random drug urine tests, and almost daily NA meetings. He worked in nonmedical service jobs for six months until his physician monitor, selected by the impaired physician program, thought he could return to medical practice, though under supervision and with continued drug testing and adherence to his recovery program.

Dr. Brown is a success story. He did not die of his addiction, develop hepatitis or get HIV from dirty needles, commit violent crimes to fund his habit, or do any (known) damage to his patients before he ran away to try to spare himself from what he needed to do. His ego functioning, when drug-free, was at the higher end, and he had the capacity for altruism, delayed gratification, and sublimation. He also had a stable marriage and a spouse who could just as well support him in recovery as try to help him elude treatment. He had a profession to return to that he loved, and colleagues invested in his returning to work and a life of contribution. He did the work of ongoing, comprehensive treatment, which included individual and group therapy, and NA. Drug testing added to his capacity to stay clean because he knew he would be caught if he used. And the prospect of returning to practice was a beacon for him to seek.

Yet Dr. Brown remains at risk to relapse. That's how it is with a substance use disorder. He will likely be in recovery for most of the lifetime ahead of him, though some people can, over time, truly put their habit behind them and regain their higher-level ego functions and the psychic resilience to rise above the addiction, never again to return to it. (This was the case for John Noble, after many years.) Recovery takes work. But it can happen with good treatment, support, purpose, the tincture of time, and keeping hope alive in patient, family, and treating clinicians.

Ego development, going from limited ego capacities in children to ego capabilities that result in generativity and dignity in adults, is a lifelong pursuit. Not only is it never over, I believe that almost everyone can move up the defensive gradient with the right kind of support and coaching. It is hard and takes time. But it is not nearly as hard or protracted as a life of interpersonal conflict, emotional distress, and foreclosed opportunities in love and work.

3

FAIL FIRST

You can always count on Americans to do the right thing—after
they've tried everything else.

—WINSTON CHURCHILL

So far we have discussed the qualities, circumstances, and outside
factors that can contribute to dangerous drug use and dependence, but what are the solutions? The United States has pursued
ineffective, costly, and deadly policies in addressing our ongoing drug crisis. We can call those policies *fail first*, borrowing
the term from the management practices often used by insurers, HMOs, managed care, and pharmacy benefit medications
with subscribers (patients in need). Often called *step therapy*, this
requires that a patient fail on one of a selected group of medications in a class before the payer will cover the cost of a more
expensive, but potentially more effective, agent.

This practice is terribly maddening to patients, families, and
doctors, who especially rebel against rules made for them by
proprietary companies driven by financial incentives. In human
costs of persistent disease and suffering, fail first can sometimes
be penny wise and pound foolish, especially in mental health.
The medical and business costs, in emergency-room visits and
hospital stays as well as absenteeism and reduced productivity,

often outweigh any savings generated by the fail-first gauntlet. Some states have limited the classes of drugs, for example the antipsychotic medications, that can be put into step-therapy programs, though that does not mean offensive delays in treatment are eliminated.

The United States has pursued a similar policy, with even greater consequences and over a longer time, against the persistent, exploding problem of drug use. Thus far, the principal policy and practice approaches to the illegal use of drugs have been control and consequences.

CONTROL

Among the many misguided endeavors by President Richard Nixon was his creation of "the War on Drugs," he being the first to use that metaphor. Not to be outdone by President Lyndon Johnson's "all-out war on human poverty," Nixon was going to take on drugs. (He had already declared war on cancer.) A combination of prohibiting drug use in the United States and military intervention in other countries, he asserted, would destroy the illegal drug trade. A "control" strategy in spades.

The casualties of this "war" have been enormous, and no evidence of its benefits has been demonstrated by any responsible government, including our own. Since President Nixon declared this war, the incarceration rate in the United States has increased by over 400 percent, resulting in the highest national incarceration rate in the world. By 1994, the war led to 1 million Americans being arrested *each year* for drugs, with about one in four arrests for marijuana possession; more recently marijuana possession has been the charge in half of the arrests in this country.

Many states implemented "three strikes" laws in the 1990s that mandated long sentences for those convicted of a crime three times. Some states instituted minimum mandatory sentences for drug trafficking, a crime often committed by people seeking to fund their addiction. By 2008, 1.5 million Americans were arrested annually for drugs, and one in three of those were incarcerated. Our prisons are filled with people of color; African Americans are sentenced to state prison thirteen times more frequently than people from other ethnic groups, making the war fundamentally racist in its effects.

Many years later, John Ehrlichman, Nixon's domestic-policy chief, admitted as much. In a recently published interview that took place in the 1990s, he said:

> You understand what I'm saying? We knew we couldn't make it illegal to be either against the [Vietnam] war or black, but by getting the public to associate the hippies with marijuana and blacks with heroin, and then criminalizing both heavily, we could disrupt those communities . . . We could arrest their leaders, raid their homes, break up their meetings, and vilify them night after night on the evening news. Did we know we were lying about the drugs? Of course we did.

By prosecuting this drug war, the Nixon team believed they would gain the white vote, especially in the South (his "Southern strategy"), and remain in the White House.

The wonderfully acted and ironic film *Elvis & Nixon* (2016) has Elvis (played brilliantly by Michael Shannon) arrange to meet with President Nixon (played deadpan by Kevin Spacey) in 1970. Elvis, "the King," more famous than the president, wants to become an undercover agent for the Feds to help break the backs of hippies and druggies, a soldier in Nixon's War on Drugs. Whatever the truth of their encounter, the photo of the two shaking hands in the Oval Office is the most requested picture in the National Archives Catalog.

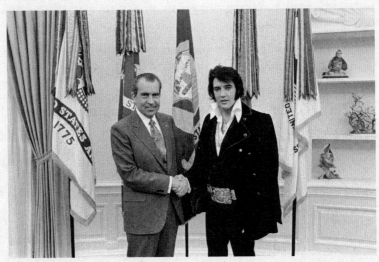

In one of the strangest White House photographs ever taken, Elvis Presley shakes hands with President Richard Nixon in the Oval Office on December 21, 1970.

Ronald Reagan too could not resist this ersatz and fabricated war, contributing to enormous rates of incarceration. The number of people in jails and prisons, largely people of color, for nonviolent drug law offenses went from fifty thousand in 1980 to more than four hundred thousand by the late nineties.

Concerns about crack cocaine were all over the press when Reagan took office in 1981. Nancy Reagan had already begun to contribute to the ill-begotten war with her Just Say No campaign. President Reagan proposed and enacted an even more militant war than Nixon. Reagan declared that "drugs were menacing our society" and asserted that his administration would achieve drug-free schools and workplaces, more vigorous law enforcement and drug interdiction, and greater public awareness.

By 1986, Reagan had passed and signed legislation that appropriated $1.7 billion to fund his War on Drugs. This included mandatory minimum prison stays for drug offenses and massive programs, at home and abroad, for crop eradication and interdiction. Public education, prevention, and rehabilitation programs had their funding *reduced*. Nancy Reagan traveled the country to speak about the dangers of drugs. Meanwhile, they both turned a blind eye to HIV/AIDS, which had begun to ravage the country.

The consequences of our history of punitive approaches to drug addiction are manifold. Public safety, particularly from incarcerating nonviolent offenders, is not significantly improved; families are broken and shattered, especially when the parents of young children are incarcerated; and recidivism is terribly high, indicating that this method of control does not effectively address the intended problems. According to the Brennan Center for Justice in New York, 39 percent of the people in US prisons are there unnecessarily since no degree of public safety is achieved. We know, as well, that two-thirds of people in correctional settings have a history of abusing drugs or alcohol or both. The Brennan Center report notes that "approximately 79% of today's prisoners suffer from either drug addiction or mental illness, and 40% suffer from both. . . . Among inmates, suicide is now the leading cause of death, accounting for 34% of deaths in 2013." Vast amounts of money are ill-spent and thus unavailable to fund prevention, alternatives to incarceration, more robust community policing, and reentry programs for prisoners upon their release.

It took until 2009 to start to move toward the light, when President Barack Obama declared that the term *War on Drugs* was not useful and would not be used by his administration. His Office of National Drug Control Policy stated, in 2011, "Drug addiction is a disease that can be successfully prevented and treated." Yet, despite these indications of forward progress, crop control, border interdiction, and state and local drug raids and seizures continue to occur, wasting billions and billions of dollars nationally and globally.

Our former president also commuted the sentences of well over one hundred people before he left office. This story was dramatized by Shruti Ganguly, one of the incredibly creative members of Fictionless, an Oscar-awarded documentary company. She directed five short films, each depicting the story of a man or woman who had been incarcerated for a nonviolent drug offense in the days of extreme mandatory sentencing. All five, two black men, two black women, and one white man, had their life or lengthy mandatory sentences commuted by President Obama, as part of his ongoing clemency for people whose punishment did not fit the crime, and who had spent most of their adult lives behind bars.

Yet there is still so much more to be done, in and out of our prison system. We know that fiction can reveal many a truth. HBO's *The Wire* (2002–08) portrayed the fictitious but alarmingly real Baltimore drug world, offering a depiction of the prison pipeline for drug offenders. The series repeatedly showed a strategy called buy-bust, in which undercover police officers buy drugs from dealers and then bust them. Their targets were invariably black. Photo ops typically ensued after a police bust, often with the display of a folding table covered with plastic-wrapped bricks of drugs and an assortment of deadly weapons and cash.

Without losing a beat, the dealers, still on the streets or incarcerated, portrayed in this series—again, fictional but very real—

would mobilize even younger boys, black adolescents too young to go to prison, to sell the very same drugs that were confiscated. What remained unchanged was the ubiquity of illegal drugs; unsafe neighborhoods; the murderous violence of the drug culture and its leaders; and the power and financial success of the dealers, who became heroes for the young to emulate, thereby inspiring the next generation of dealers and users.

"Follow the money" is the other fuel, besides covert racism and political propaganda, that propels the engine of the drug wars. To see the futility of drug-control endeavors, read Tom Wainwright's illuminating book *Narconomics* (2016). He meticulously shows how supply-side interventions, such as crop control, interdiction, and buy-bust, are as useless in Colombia and Mexico as they are on the streets of Baltimore, New York, and London. Wainwright, now UK editor for *The Economist*, had been the magazine's correspondent in Mexico for years. The only major form of "news" was drugs, the cartels, and their murderous ways, which became his material for *Narconomics*.

Wainwright reveals how the hundreds of billions of dollars spent on efforts to control drug supplies in recent years have failed miserably to reduce cartel production and the use of illegal drugs, which are consumed by *250 million people* worldwide. The heart of Wainwright's argument is that the relentless focus on supply-side efforts to reduce illegal drug use has proven useless and that a demand-side approach would likely yield far more success. His examples about supply-side drug economics are compelling.

For example, he writes that the world economies spend an estimated US$100 billion annually to combat the cartels, $20 billion federally in the United States. Crop eradication and interdiction, favorite tactics in the drug war, have almost zero financial impact on cartel costs. Even when growers have had to produce twice the amount of cocaine, for instance, the buyers (i.e., the cartels) pay them no additional money; the price at the end of the line stays the same, on the streets of London and New York, thereby not adversely affecting sales. This is because the cartels have what he calls a monopsony, in which only one, or one predominant, purchaser exists, who then dictates the price it will pay: either sell to us at the price we set or you get nothing.

Take cocaine as an example. Even doubling the sale price of the coca leaf in the mountains, were that to happen absent a monopsony, would increase the cost to a street purchaser by less than 1 percent. Why? Because of the economics of the supply chain, the sequence by which a commodity is produced and distributed. The principal costs are not for the product, but for the multitude of illegal and expensive steps from the field to the nasal mucosa of the consumer. Wainwright likens efforts to reduce user (end-point) purchases by raising the price of coca leaves to trying to increase the price of expensive paintings by increasing the price of paint. He argues that the way to destroy the drug business is to cut the heart out of its revenues by reducing consumer demand. That might work because, as has been said, "it's the economy, stupid."

Control strategies have simply not done the job: drug delivery and access go unfettered, with only momentary interruptions, while the prices users pay are barely impacted and drug use goes unabated. Yet, the principal strategies for drug control pronounced by the Trump administration are to "build a wall" and "get tough on users and dealers." Should all control efforts be suspended? While I greatly support decriminalizing possession of limited quantities of drugs, that is different from controlling such substances as synthetic marijuana (K2 or spice) and crack cocaine and crystal meth. Those are examples of drugs so damaging that we need more than demand reduction alone. But what we have not parsed out is which drugs and which control efforts should be sustained and which should be stopped, and then repurpose that money for prevention and treatment efforts. Budget woes at the federal and state levels are going to preclude sufficient new money for demand reduction, for prevention and treatment, and for us to succeed the funds must come from somewhere.

The metaphor *the War on Drugs* presupposes an enemy outside our borders or a civil uprising threatening the future of the nation. This is where the metaphor—applied to drugs as well as poverty and cancer—fails us from the very start. There is no external enemy.

Drugs are what people with addictions use; they are not armies at the gate. Addiction is "self-induced changes in neuro-transmission that result in problem behavior." Rather than facing an enemy, we have a powerful convergence of biology and social circumstances, the interplay of nature and nurture, that produces addictions—spanning alcohol, drugs, and a variety of compulsive behaviors such as gambling, video games, and some sexual disorders. How can we prosecute a war on human problems? The conditions to win such a "war" simply do not exist.

But the fatal consequences of the ongoing drug war are epidemic and visible.

In the film *The Untouchables*, the salty veteran Irish street cop Jim Malone (Sean Connery) takes a moment to advise the green, ambitious FBI agent Eliot Ness (Kevin Costner) after an eruption of deadly violence. Malone says, "You wanna know how to get Capone? They pull a knife, you pull a gun. They send one of yours to the hospital, you send one of theirs to the morgue. That's the Chicago way." But it is more than the Chicago way, though that city has certainly been a bleak poster child for violence. Just across the border in Mexico, cartels—such as Los Zetas, Knights Templar, and Sinaloa—enforce order and maintain their market shares through violence, including beheadings, torture, and mass killings. Homicides in Mexico peaked at almost twenty-three thousand a year in 2011, dropped to a bit over fifteen thousand in 2014, and are now on the rebound. Murder pays. And we all suffer, drug users and nonusers alike, from the policies of control and incarceration that have characterized the US approach to addiction for much of our long history.

CONSEQUENCES

Doctor: "Joe, you're fifty pounds overweight. That's starting to give you diabetes and high blood pressure. Plus, it's one of the reasons your knees hurt so much. You need to lose that weight."

Joe: "You're right, Doc. I'll do it."

When Joe leaves his doctor's office, he leaves his good intentions behind as if returning a magazine to a table in the waiting room. The next time he has a doctor's appointment, he is reluctant to go, feeling ashamed. When he does go, the doctor-patient pas de deux is unchanged. The doctor once again exhorts Joe to lose weight. Joe knows the consequences of being overweight, but that is not enough to mobilize him to act.

I heard an apocryphal story many years ago before the use of seat belts became common. The public service ads and threats of fines were not getting good traction, nor was negative advertising, showing people in hospital beds or coffins. The story goes, however, that one advertisement was different. It depicted an adorable child in the back seat admonishing her dad to buckle up. That worked. Estimates are that today over 1 million lives have been saved by the use of seat belts.

The use of children to promote safety in adults, who can't as a group seem to abide by simple and effective rules for their own welfare, has migrated to another grim problem: accidental shootings by youth with their parents' handguns. When the tables were turned on the parents, hammering them with how they might be endangering their children, they paid more attention.

When I speak about how effective drugs, legal and illegal, are in achieving their desired effects on how a person feels, thinks, and acts, almost invariably the response is "But they cause cancer" or "They can lead to HIV infection" or "They destroy a person's brain—and their lives." Of course they can and sometimes do, especially if they are impure and used in unhygienic and unsafe ways. Cigarette smoking and vaping are always harmful, always. But while some limited effect is achieved by putting big black or red letters spelling out CANCER or CIGARETTES KILL on cigarette packs, what has worked far better has been making smokers pariahs in their own families and communities.

There's a joke about a man going into a pharmacy and asking in a clear, loud voice for a package of condoms, then whispering a request for a pack of cigarettes. Social values and family influences matter, not exhorting people to not do what they already know they shouldn't do.

Risky behaviors in youth (and even adults) also don't respond particularly strongly to admonitions, such as against sexually transmitted diseases, injuries, unwanted pregnancy, texting while driving, sexting, and the development of anorexia nervosa. Yet, emphasizing the negative consequences of alcohol, tobacco, and drugs has been the second major strategy in dealing with drug use and abuse. A variant, also ineffective, is having uniformed policemen come to schools and warn students about the laws against drug use and the misery of prison. They may feel good for the moment, especially for educators desperate to help, but these warnings also don't work.

Rattling on about consequences is akin to jousting with windmills, being unable to see the world as it is, just like Don Quixote. What we need is a Sancho Panza, a fellow companion who comments wisely and with humor and irony, to allow us to change the dialogue.

The disconnect between information, in this case cautionary details, and action is massive. If we all acted with reason, in our self-interest, my profession would not need to exist. But it does, and business remains brisk.

Ongoing campaigns, public service announcements, and school education programs that teach youth the consequences of their actions have been just as fixed and ineffective as efforts to control the use of drugs. Some youth do appreciate, it's true, the difference between experimenting with drugs and becoming regular users, for instance, or the importance of staying away from the "needle barrier." But prevention programs in schools have relied on adults, whom adolescents are more apt to rebel against than listen to; some programs have recently started to use other youth, peers, to deliver the demand-reduction message, which is an improvement. But still youth face the intrinsic limitations on controlling their behaviors that, in time, the maturation of their brains will provide.

Modern neuroscience has proven that the human brain does not fully myelinate—surround the massive number of connecting fibers among brain nerve cells with a fatty insulating substance, thereby enhancing conduction—until the early to middle twenties, sometimes later for males. The myelin enables our brains to work more effectively, especially our frontal lobes, where judgment derives from. Think of the times you or a friend asked teenagers to do something, remember something, control their impulses, cap their emotions, or even just cap the toothpaste. Something is missing in their heads, and it is called myelin. The absence of myelin is a neurological reason for not permitting voting until age eighteen and making the sale of tobacco and alcohol (and cannabis) subject to age restrictions, which I think are examples of selective control measures we should sustain.

That is not to say, however, that once humans have passed their third decade on earth they become exemplars of healthy and decent behavior. They have a better chance at it, but as we see every day, it is no foregone conclusion. We do know, though, that people whose adolescence was spent under the sway of substances lose those years of psychological and emotional development and remain rooted in more juvenile ways of thinking and being.

Bearing down on consequences is a puritan and punitive approach to controlling behaviors that time has shown—as has the growth of substance use, abuse, and overdoses—not worthy of the amount of effort and resources it has consumed. It's not valueless, but it's just not enough if we are to alter the trajectory and popularity of substance use in this country.

A technique that originated in the substance-treatment community years ago has now become popular in managing chronic physical conditions such as diabetes, hypertension, and heart disease, and habit disorders such as smoking and overeating, in general medicine and primary-care settings, as well as in mental health and addiction clinical services. It is called motivational interviewing (MI) or motivational enhancement (ME).

People don't smoke because it makes them smell bad or gives

them cancer. Painful relationships don't persist because of the disappointments and grief they generate. Troubling habits of all sorts endure because of *what they do for us*. Motivation to change can come from a person's getting more out of changing than staying where he or she may be, which is the basis of motivational interviewing.

Motivational interviewing is nonjudgmental. There is no saying a person is bad or his or her behaviors are shameful. Nor does it allow people to emotionally beat up on themselves, self-flagellating with negative, abusive comments. Quite the opposite: MI starts by recognizing that a person is doing something for powerful reasons. The best ideas that emerge in MI come from the patient, in a trusting relationship with the clinician.

In another section of this book, we will look at other ways to change damaging habits, especially addictions, based on the neuroscience of behavior.

We must employ more than exhortation, more than shame and nagging, to help a person live a healthier and more rewarding life. MI is but one example, as are other cognitive techniques, family supports, medication-assisted treatments, recovery groups, exercise, and a variety of useful mind-body approaches including yoga, slow breathing, mindfulness, and meditation. The alternatives to "accentuating the negative" work far better.

PART TWO

HOW TO SUCCEED

4

AN OUNCE OR A TON?

. . . let us try to offer help before we have to offer therapy. That is to say, let's see if we can't prevent being ill by trying to offer a love of prevention before illness.

—MAYA ANGELOU

A new flood was predicted and nothing could prevent it. In three days, the waters would wipe out the world.

The Dalai Lama appeared on worldwide media and pleaded with humanity to follow Buddhist teachings to find nirvana in the wake of the disaster.

The pope issued a similar message, saying, "It is still not too late to accept Jesus."

The chief rabbi of Jerusalem took a slightly different approach. "My people," he said, "we have three days to learn how to live underwater."

—YIDDISH JOKE

To recognize the salience of prevention, we need to think of it not as an "ounce" but something closer to a "ton."

For twenty years, from 1989 to 2008, California invested $2.4 billion of its tax dollars from cigarette sales in what was called the California Tobacco Control Program. The money was spent on efforts to reduce smoking, including funding community coalitions that sought to implement no-smoking policies and practices, as well as on informing public-media campaigns.

An analysis of this investment performed by the University of California, San Francisco, considered changes in smoking prevalence, cigarette consumption, and health-care costs: $134 billion was saved by the program, producing a 5,500 percent return on investment (ROI) from reductions in the cost of treatment of smoking-related illnesses.

Youth are especially prone to using alcohol, drugs, and tobacco. Experimentation is normative, as is risk taking and the drive to defy authority as a path to independence. Moreover, the capacity of the brains of youth to control their impulses and behaviors is biologically limited because, as noted earlier, myelination is still under way. Finally, peer and media influences are everywhere, especially those pro-drug messages in music, TV, and movies. We can expect substance use and will likely continue to see it widely. Our collective work and responsibility is to limit its damages.

Three levels of action, or intervention, have characterized scientific writings on prevention, including prevention of behavioral health conditions like addictions. This construction builds on public-health principles that consider a population—an aggregate group—of people, some at risk of a condition and some not. These definitions are described here more specifically for populations of youth.

Universal programs aim to reach all youth, whether they are at known risk or not. These are also known as *primary, universal prevention. Selective programs* aim to reach youth exposed to known and high levels of risk for a condition, but who have not yet become symptomatic. These are also known as primary prevention for at-risk groups. *Indicated programs* are those that aim to serve youth showing indicia of early behavioral health problems, and are sometimes called secondary prevention.

As we dig more deeply, an understanding of prevention is nicely illuminated by a model that divides individuals according to their unique characteristics in two key ways: risk factors and protective factors. These are the yin and yang of prevention.

Risk factors are those environmental, familial, or individual elements that carry greater risk for promoting a health problem, in this case a substance use disorder. Protective factors, similarly, exist outside and inside all of us and can reduce the potential for problem substance use and abuse. Risk and protective factors vary from one person to another and can change over a person's life.

Adding to this perspective, which is useful in policy and program development, we can consider risk and protective factors by "domain"—namely, wherein the locus of the problem or intervention may principally be located.

Risk and Protective Factors for Substance Use Disorders

Risk Factors	Domain	Protective Factors
Early Aggressive Behavior	Individual	Impulse Control
Lack of Parental Supervision	Family	Parental Monitoring
Substance Abuse	Peer	Academic Competence
Drug Availability	School	Antidrug Use Policies
Poverty	Community	Strong Neighborhood Attachment

One way to understand risk and protective factors, essential in preventing drug abuse, is by the domain they affect.

Let's go back to the life of Billie Holiday. Is there a risk factor she did not have? Is there a blessed protective factor she enjoyed, in any or all of these domains? She didn't stand a chance: she was dead at forty-four, along the way having been a high "user" of health-care and correctional facilities, with their attendant costs.

In an interview, I was once asked, "If you could wave a wand and do one thing that would make a world of future difference for youth and their physical, mental, and addictive health, and the avoidance of time spent in jails and prisons, what would that be?" My mind did not go to some great scientific discovery, as welcome as that would be, but rather to what was destroying the health and welfare of so many children and adolescents now, and where action could be taken today.

My answer was to eliminate ACEs. ACEs are "adverse childhood experiences," which can usher in a lifetime of misfortune—and frequently then pass troubles on to succeeding generations. These are events beyond young people's control. Through no choice of their own these youth are subject to powerful stressors that adversely impact their minds and bodies.

The principal types of ACEs are abuse, neglect, and seriously troubled households. Specifically, ACEs include emotional, physical, and sexual abuse; emotional and physical neglect; and homes that have domestic violence, mental and/or substance use disorders, parental separation or divorce; or a family member who is incarcerated. ACEs occur before a child reaches the age of eighteen—but their effects are painfully enduring.

Luisa Gomez, age fourteen, who lives with her grandmother in Spanish Harlem, is pregnant and failing in school. She is obese, smokes, and is showing metabolic evidence of insulin insensitivity, a precursor to adult-onset diabetes. She has been diagnosed with depression and has already taken an overdose of tranquilizers after a disappointment with her boyfriend, using pills she found in a friend's bathroom cabinet. She was raised in a series of foster homes from age five until eleven, placed there after she was sexually abused by her stepfather and because her mother, addicted to crack cocaine, was unable to care for her. Her father had abandoned her mother shortly after Luisa was born. Her grandmother is infirm, and Luisa takes more care of her than the grandmother does of Luisa. Her pregnancy was the result of unprotected sex and the underlying need to prove that she was desirable to boys. It is unclear who is the father of Luisa's child. Her future looks dismal, with few skills, limited education, minimal adult support, and a body and mind already suffering from the consequences of a host of adverse childhood experiences.

Sadly, there are many Luisas (and their male counterparts) throughout our country. Their suffering and burden to society are vast, likely unmeasurable.

What is so troubling about ACEs is that they are additive. One is bad enough, but four, five, or more are a powerful prescription for illness and despair, often by adolescence. ACEs can lead youth in this or any other country to such problems, among many others, as alcohol and drug abuse; depression; heart, lung, and liver diseases; STDs; intimate-partner violence; smoking, especially at an early age; suicide attempts; and unintended pregnancies. As the number of ACEs youth experience increases, so too does their risk for multiple consequences.

ACEs seem to do their damage in two principal ways: first, by inducing a chronic stress response in the brain, and thus body, which lowers immunity to disease and is instrumental in the development of a variety of mental and physical illnesses such as depression and PTSD—as well as limiting the capacity to recover from them. Second, they also do damage in the long term, producing effects such as cigarette smoking, alcohol and drug abuse, and unprotected sex. The combined results of chronic stress and risky behaviors induce a host of diseases and social problems, often by adolescence or young adulthood. Diseases and disorders mount, limiting functioning and quality of life and producing disability and early death.

It is because of the prevalence of ACEs and because of their impact on our youth that I answered the interviewer's question the way I did.

Prevention of ACEs is no small feat. But there are ways to make a difference, now. And the payoff might even exceed the return on investment seen in California's anti-tobacco campaign. Frederick Douglass said, "It is easier to build strong children than to repair broken men."

A couple examples of proven approaches to ACEs and childhood trauma and behavioral problems come to mind.

The first step must be prevention of the consequences of childhood abuse, neglect, and troubled homes, which remains elusive despite its importance. I asked Laurie Miller Brotman, PhD, a colleague at NYU and a friend, to give us an example of how a family beset with adverse childhood experiences was helped by ParentCorps, her community-based intervention that is delivered as an enhancement to pre-K programs.

Graciela is a married woman in her early forties who has struggled with anxiety since immigrating to New York as a teenager. She experienced both sexual harassment in her factory job and severe postpartum depression after the birth of Jaden, her only child. Jaden was four years old when a teacher at his pre-K program told his mom about ParentCorps. Graciela struggled to respond to Jaden's behavior at home and was afraid to tell anyone how out of control she felt. She felt isolated and was sure she was failing as a mother.

The social worker at the pre-K program helped Graciela garner the courage to walk through the door of the first of fourteen conveniently scheduled ParentCorps sessions. She was hesitant and unsure if it would be helpful. She had tried everything she could think of to calm Jaden and prevent his tantrums and screaming.

She was surprised when the ParentCorps facilitator, the same trusted social worker who'd brought her there, talked with her and the other parents about their lives, what they valued, and their goals for their children. Graciela was asked to think about her own upbringing—what she wanted to repeat as a mother and what she wanted to leave behind.

The most powerful experience for Graciela was hearing from other parents about their own struggles, as well as learning what behaviors were "normal" for four-year-olds. She was scared about her son and how often she and her husband fought about how to respond to him. But she came to feel safe at the meetings with the other parents; she was eager to learn about how to create routines such as helping Jaden go to bed on time and stay in his own bed all night. She also learned how to help her son cope with frustration and anger.

As Graciela went home each week and put her new knowledge into practice, she began to see results. Her son's behavior improved rapidly. Within a few weeks, and with additional support from the social worker, Jaden's tantrums ceased altogether. He began sleeping in his own bed all night, a huge accomplishment and a relief to his parents. These parenting successes with Jaden had ripple effects throughout the family, easing tension between Graciela and her husband and reducing Graciela's anxiety. She started to trust her instincts as a mother and experimented with ways to bring the concepts she was learning to other parts of her life.

Brotman and her team at the Center for Early Childhood Health and Development are partnering with the NYC Division of Early Childhood Education to bring ParentCorps to fifty pre-K programs and have plans to help families create safe, nurturing, and predictable environments in the classroom and at home in three hundred additional programs. All told, their 1,850 programs serve seventy thousand children annually.

A second example is the enduring program Big Brothers Big Sisters, operating since 1904. Their tagline is "Millions of children need a caring adult role model," which seems to me to be a modest underestimate. Their theory of change is that the regular presence of a caring adult is a powerful antidote to youth engaging in risky, even dangerous, behaviors, and to keeping their focus on school and healthy relationships.

Big Brothers Big Sisters seeks out youth at risk: those living in foster care, in dangerous neighborhoods, and in homes riddled with domestic violence or drug use, and these already having encounters with the juvenile justice system. These are kids apt to be swallowed up by the chaos and destruction of the environments they live in, through no choice of their own. The youth are not only attached to their big brother or sister, but are also exposed to art, music, sports, education, and community organizations where contribution is the prevailing ethos for them to learn.

These are but two of many examples of how prevention and early intervention can keep so many youth from lives of disruption, addiction, incarceration, and despair.

Other wonderful examples include home visits to first-time

moms by nurses; programs such as Positive Parenting and the Incredible Years; as well as pediatric and primary-care screening and early intervention for depression and substance use problems in youth; and trauma-focused treatment programs for youth already showing problems. We have alternatives, but so far their adoption is terribly limited.

Again, consider Billie Holiday. Her mother was addicted to narcotics, her father missing. As a youth, her community was a brothel. Violence pummeled her, from rape at age ten to ongoing abuse by her pimp-husband. She was jailed, sent to reform school, and punished. By the time she was an adolescent she was homeless, drinking heavily, and en route to a heroin habit.

But not all those subject to ACEs draw such a profoundly miserable deal. Even for those who do, children and adolescents with a decent measure of resilience, self-control, and support can change the trajectory of their lives—but the odds at first are against them. They need help, as do their families.

Returning to the nosology of universal, selected, and indicated aspects of prevention, with a focus on adolescence, there are many ways to facilitate change, though they are not as often employed as they could be.

On a *universal level*, a fine and demonstrably effective example is LifeSkills Training (LST). LST curricula are available for elementary schools (grades three to six); middle or junior high schools (grades six to eight or seven to nine); and high schools (grades nine or ten). For example, LST can be delivered for three years in middle schools. Students are taught essential, usually previously underdeveloped skills, such as problem solving and decision making, which help these youth resist peers and media encouraging drug use—also called drug-resistance skills—as well as coping mechanisms and methods to manage stress and anxiety. Self-esteem and self-control typically improve. LST shows sustained effects with preventing tobacco, alcohol, and marijuana use as well as binge drinking.

Another *universal approach* is exemplified by the family-based Strengthening Families Program: For Parents and Youth 10–14. Provided in rural areas, this program helps parents build the skills to manage a family, communicate in positive ways, improve relationships with their children, and support academic and extracurricular activities. There is considerable flexibility in where and when services are delivered, and babysitting, transportation, and meals help with engagement and ongoing family participation.

A *selective-level intervention* for high-risk schools and youth is the Project Towards No Drug Abuse (TND), though it has also spread to some schools and students not clearly at risk—unless we consider all school youth at risk, which has some face validity. In working with students fourteen to nineteen years of age, the goal is to help them resist substance use. TND is delivered in twelve forty-to-fifty-minute lessons; it too teaches social skills and decision making, as well as aiming to improve student motivation to stay clean. There are group discussions, role-playing exercises, and videos.

An example of an *indicated approach* is the Brief Alcohol Screening and Intervention for College Students (BASICS) program. BASICS is directed toward college students already showing evidence of heavy drinking, and who are at risk for alcohol-related problems such as accidents, poor class attendance, failure to meet deadlines on assignments, sexual assault, and violent behavior. BASICS, done in two one-hour meetings with an online assessment between the two, seeks to help students reduce alcohol consumption and thereby decrease its consequences.

The time is right, as well, for introducing and broadly disseminating Screening, Brief Intervention, and Referral to Treatment

(SBIRT) for youth. This can be done at universal (primary-care/pediatric), selective (school- and community-program), and indicated (emergency-room and juvenile-justice) levels. SBIRT for some, but not all, affected youth is becoming an essential element of behavioral health–care services in general-, primary-, and family-medicine practices. Teenagers at risk or showing evidence of alcohol and drug abuse—for instance, accidents, missing school or failing in class, risky behaviors, trouble with the law, worrisome changes in friend groups, frequent medical problems without a clear physical condition—in pediatric, primary-care, or emergency services are asked as few as two questions. The first question is about friends' drinking, an early-warning sign that is highly associated with the youth's current or future substance use and is often more effective than asking the youth directly about himself. The second question is about the youth him- or herself, directly inquiring about frequency of substance use.

The American Academy of Pediatrics, in 2011, recommended substance screening as a "routine" part of adolescent health care.

SBIRT has varied approaches for youth ages nine to eleven, eleven to fourteen, and fourteen to eighteen (where the patient question is asked before the question about friends). It is a good example of secondary prevention, that is, the detection and treatment of a condition before it advances and becomes more fixed. While some youth respond to the primary-care doctor's concern and counseling, others do not and will require "referral to treatment," the last part of SBIRT's name. Some physicians are reluctant to adopt SBIRT because they worry about their capacity to adequately refer their patients. Shortages of substance use disorder services can be legion, particularly when crossing the chasm from a medical-care setting to behavioral health care. There's also the problem of both sites getting adequately reimbursed, the federal Parity

Act and its Health and Human Services regulations notwithstanding. The concern of these doctors adds more voices to the call for greater access to and coverage of quality care for youth (and adults) experiencing every level of problems with alcohol and drugs.

I would be remiss not to touch on community-based approaches to prevention. As a rule, the more of these mobilized, the more effective their collective impact—in academic, family, and also community settings. Community approaches also include media campaigns and community organizations (such as the Y, Big Brothers Big Sisters, and local gyms), as well as faith-based settings and programs. Public-policy initiatives can also be community based, such as sanctions for servers who sell alcohol to minors, regulations to limit the number of bars and liquor stores, and aggressive sobriety stops for drivers.

A great many other examples of prevention of alcohol and drug problems exist. As with other sections in this book, I am offering illustrations—not a textbook or an encyclopedia of materials. I hope I have begun to show how much has been done, and just how much work remains.

PRINCIPLES OF PREVENTION

A set of critical principles underlie public-health approaches to prevention. In considering and selecting from available methods, it is useful to see if any given prevention approach meets the recognized principles that forecast success. They include:

- Family, school, primary-care, or community-serving locations
- Early screening and detection

- Identifying and intervening with the social determinants of addiction (e.g., ACEs)
- The prominent use, for adolescents, of peers
- Ready access to equitable, affordable, effective, comprehensive treatment
- Relentless use of data to measure the problem(s) selected, to monitor the effectiveness of efforts, and to check for continuous quality improvement
- The capacity of a program to "scale up," or become commonly present throughout an area
- Insistent demand for adoption of policies that capture savings (from health care, social welfare, and corrections) and use of those savings to further invest in prevention and treatment

I hope no one thinks that after all my years of developing, implementing, and running services, clinically and governmentally, that I imagine that delivering on a prevention agenda is easy. It most certainly is not. But if the Wright brothers, Jonas Salk, Watson and Crick, Marie Curie, Nelson Mandela, Martin Luther King, and countless others had been cowed by complexity and resistance, we would still want for their discoveries and the impact they have had on society.

5

MEANINGFUL ENGAGEMENT AND ALTERNATIVES

"Healing," / Papa would tell me, / "is not a science, / but the intuitive art / of wooing Nature."
—W. H. AUDEN, "THE ART OF HEALING"

When you come upon a wall, throw your hat over it, and then go get your hat.
—IRISH PROVERB

Every society, for as long as we can discern, has used psychoactive drugs. The purposes have varied, including facilitating religious rites, spiritual journeys, and coming-of-age transitions; delivering stamina and easing bodily pain; lubricating social encounters; and the not-so-mere pleasure of taking leave, however transiently, from life's slings and arrows, from the psychic pains that are part of being human.

As I mentioned before, the Inuit had been the exception until explorers, white men given to liquid spirits, introduced them to alcohol. Now there are no exceptions. Some experts contend that this is evidence that achieving altered states of feeling and consciousness are a basic human drive, like hunger and sex.

Societal acceptance, or not, of the use of psychoactive substances tends to have far more to do with the culture and ideology of the people than the drug itself. History too has been a factor. Opium, as noted earlier, was used extensively by Chinese immigrant workers when they built the American railroad tracks. Now opioids are at the core of the war on drugs. Cocaine was once an ingredient in a popular wine (Vin Mariani) as well as in Coca-Cola. Alcohol went through the drunken policy failure of Prohibition and is now a major drug of choice, widely marketed in this country—thank you, Anheuser-Busch, Coors, and other beverage companies. Marijuana has been particularly batted around over the ages from legal to illegal and to legal again, with recreational cannabis now legalized in eight states and DC (with more en route); and more than half of the states allow for its medical prescription. Take a walk down the seaside path that runs along Venice Beach, California, and for a small fee a doctor will write a recommendation for cannabis that you can have filled then and there, continuing your stroll under the influence. (Though I wonder if this business will last now that California has legalized recreational marijuana.)

Many countries are more liberal about psychoactive drugs than is the United States. While marijuana is "illegal" in the Netherlands, about every block in Amsterdam has "coffee shops" that serve a pot of coffee as well as smokable pot. Portugal has fully decriminalized drugs. Vancouver, Canada, has safe injection sites for using heroin, and the young, progressive prime minister of Canada has now made heroin available by prescription. Switzerland and the United Kingdom as well allow for the prescription of heroin. In Uruguay, marijuana can be purchased at pharmacies by those twenty-one or older. There are other examples, of course, but my aim is to show how varied, even fickle, policies, laws, and practices can be, worldwide. This is also evidence not only that psychoactive drug use is ubiquitous, but that it will go on whether we legalize (or decriminalize) it or not, prescribe it or not, tax and regulate it or not, or simply turn a blind eye, hoping to ignore its consumption by scores of millions of people.

As a public-health doctor, I am very aware that access to a substance is generally associated with its increased use. Yet for many psychoactive substances that has not proven to be the case in a variety of countries, and it remains to be seen what will happen with legal marijuana in the United States. Moreover, as Johann Hari has pointed out, where legal use has increased, the harms associated with drug use have decreased, including over-dose deaths, HIV/AIDS, criminal behaviors, and racially discriminatory incarcerations. Furthermore, money not wasted on pursuit of criminals and correctional remedies can be critically repurposed for prevention and treatment.

I am *not* a proponent for across-the-board legalization of all psychoactive substances. They are simply too varied in their chemistry, their dangers to body and brain, and their impact on families, health, and community. I am not a proponent, either, of further legalizing recreational marijuana until we are more fully informed by the natural experiments now going on. We need to better learn how to protect teenage brains, ensure the reliability of the dose and quality of the drugs distributed, and learn a lot more about how to manage the finances of this expensive-to-regulate drug, as well as get away from the fully cash transactions that federal illegalization has produced. The first person you see upon entering a legal recreational marijuana dispensary is a security guard with a sidearm and a Kevlar vest.

We need more time to sort through the data from an increasing number of countries and states to know which substances can be relatively safely and effectively legalized, and for what ages and with what regulatory controls. But this is not to say that we should continue the romance with law and order, control and interdiction, and criminalization of what every culture uses and will continue to use.

The basic premise of this book is that people use drugs for a purpose. They work. Patterns of use can be light or heavy, periodic or steady, recreational or compulsive, legal or illicit, safe or not—dependent on prevailing views and ideologies about any given drug as well as the personality of those taking them (set and setting, once again). But drugs are winning the drug war. Better to make love than war, which means, here, first appreciating the purposes drugs serve and then offering alternatives—either to prevent psychoactive drug use or to enable people to move from the potential harm of illicit drug use and its unsafe practices, medically and criminally, to alternative ways of changing how they feel and think. We can offer humans and societies ways to achieve different altered states of consciousness that are safer, healthier, and more socially acceptable.

Roger Ebert began his career as a film critic in 1967, writing for the *Chicago Sun-Times*. Soon after, he lectured and taught film at the University of Chicago. In 1975, he won the Pulitzer Prize for Criticism and began hosting, with Gene Siskel, one of the most entertaining and smart film-reviewing TV shows, famous for its thumbs-up and thumbs-down ratings. The show endured, including a move to PBS and then Disney.

Ebert had been a heavy drinker in his early years, but quit in 1979 at age thirty-seven with the help of AA. He was obese and some years later settled into a routine of ten thousand steps a day, an exercise regimen that could do us all some good. He ate more nutritiously as well, and had a good marriage, at age fifty, to trial attorney Charlie "Chaz" Hammelsmith. Exercise, diet, and a trusting, supportive relationship were the elements that propelled and enriched his life.

At age sixty, Ebert was diagnosed with a rare form of thyroid cancer, requiring first surgery on this gland, then on his local salivary glands, and then radiation. Misfortune did not leave him, and a few years later, following further surgery for cancer of the jaw, he had a carotid artery bleed, a life-threatening event. He was left disfigured and unable to speak, or to eat or drink normally.

But he was resilient. He had purpose, love, support, and determination on his side. After an extended absence he returned to work, first communicating through his wife and then through print media. His health, unfortunately, continued to decline, and he died at the age of seventy.

Upon his death, President Barack Obama wrote, "Roger was the movies. . . . [He could capture] the unique power of the movies to take us somewhere magical. . . . The movies won't be the same without Roger." Robert Redford described Ebert as "one of the great champions of freedom of artistic expression." Oprah Winfrey remarked that his death was the "end of an era," and Steven Spielberg said that Ebert's "reviews went far deeper than simply thumbs up or thumbs down. He wrote with passion through a real knowledge of film and film history, and in doing so, helped many movies find their audiences. . . . [He] put television criticism on the map."

This formerly obese, lonely, and alcoholic man found the alternatives he needed to leave some pretty big problems behind and make a life of relationships, creativity, and contribution.

*   *   *

Following are some examples of the alternatives that are available to everyone.

EXERCISE AND SPORTS

Among the least controversial, the most lauded, of alternatives is exercise. There is *one thing* that humans can do that will significantly and salubriously alter their mood, sense of well-being, and cardiac, metabolic, and mental functioning and deliver a longer, healthier life—namely, regular aerobic exercise. Ten thousand steps a day on your smartphone, Apple Watch, or Fitbit; running; cycling; swimming; ballroom dancing; or playing tennis, basketball, or racquetball are just a few of the ways to do it.

Some people will need the support of a partner, a group, a gym, or a trainer. It doesn't matter how; what matters is exercising, getting your heart and respiration rate up and your muscles pumping blood, for several hours a week at least. For the record, and for careful readers, if people are harming themselves with tobacco, immoderate drinking, and unsafe drug use, that will bury the benefits of exercise. But exercise is the healthiest, most affordable, and most available alternative we have to psychoactive substances. Since a teenager, exercise has been my drug of choice. I have the sports injuries to prove it. I wish I could still play basketball and singles tennis, but walking, hiking, elliptical and cycling machines, and swimming will just have to do as I grow older.

Aerobic exercise creates additional arterial channels in the heart to protect us from atherosclerotic disease, which compromises vital cardiac blood flow, and has also been shown to be the most effective way to slow down any intrinsic progression toward Alzheimer's disease. To add to its wonders, strenuous exercise releases brain endorphins, our natural opioids that reduce pain and evoke a feeling of well-being: the runner's high.

For youth, active-sports programs are one of the better preventatives against teenage drug use and abuse. Not only do sports highly engage their time and energy and provide a departure from whatever difficulties they may be experiencing, but a commitment to sports is a strong deterrent to using drugs, a good way to say no when approached by peers or dealers.

I would advise anyone to start slow but not to hesitate to make exercise part of his or her life. To enjoy and reap its benefits, individuals don't have to be athletes—just physically active people.

MEDITATION, YOGA, YOGIC BREATHING, AND MINDFULNESS

Eastern yogis and gurus have for millennia employed various forms of meditation and breathing techniques to achieve inner states of calm and peace and to remarkably alter their autonomic (fight-or-flight) nervous system. Dramatic reductions in heart rate, temperature, and respiration have been achieved by some mystics and probably by Houdini as well, since he was able to survive being locked up underwater for lengthy periods (how he unlocked the chains is beyond me).

Meditation and yogic breathing—a form of slow breathing, five to six breaths a minute with gentle resistance on exhalation—

can enable us to regulate bodily functions previously thought inaccessible to our conscious efforts and also have a profound effect on the mind's executive functions (e.g., focus, sustained concentration, short-term memory, and sequencing of actions) and our capacity for awareness of ourselves and others.

We possess, by virtue of human consciousness, the capacity to know we exist and to hold a sense of self, of identity, of personhood. Humans are self-aware. But awareness is limited and can grow dimmer with the passage of time and the blinders of everyday existence. The desire to both expand awareness and, paradoxically, lose the sense of self to a more universal experience is particularly sought after by adolescents and young adults.

Psychoactive drugs can be quick and efficient ways to alter consciousness. Meditation is another means, though it takes effort—effort until it becomes effortless. Many schools of meditation exist. Some rely on a mantra, others on breathing rhythms and focus, still others on observing the mind and breath and a relationship with a teacher, as does Zen. Often meditation is coupled with a yoga practice.

Transcendental Meditation was popularized in the United States many decades ago. I learned Transcendental Meditation while in medical school and used it on and off until I began to practice yogic breathing some years ago. Once, while volunteering for a study on brain-wave activity while in medical school, I had my electroencephalograph, or EEG, readings taken while practicing Transcendental Meditation. I was delighted to learn that, compared to my normal EEG reading, my alpha waves—a type of brain waves produced during peaceful relaxation, possibly playing a role in effective brain-circuit activities—were particularly prominent during my meditation.

Many meditation centers, experts, and even online services teach meditation. It is highly accessible, affordable, and generally readily learned. But as with exercise, repetition with meditation is the road to its nirvana. Changing our consciousness, which can get stuck in familiar patterns from the endless repetition of existing, takes some doing. But it has been done for thousands of years. Meditation, yoga, and breathing techniques are psychoactive-substance alternatives that are safe and, over time, effective in supplying the human appetite with experiences beyond the everyday, the mundane, and the dysphoric.

The practice of mindfulness appears to have been derived from the Buddhist practice of *sati*, which means "awareness." Through mindfulness, people can gain awareness of the present moment, at once also recognizing and accepting their feelings, thoughts, and bodily sensations. The practitioner may eventually come to appreciate that all feeling states are transient, transitory, and will pass. This knowledge is invaluable to people who are flooded by feelings that paralyze them or compel them to act and is highly useful in resisting the cravings experienced by substance-dependent individuals.

Mindfulness has been used for stress reduction, as a meditative technique, and as an essential component of dialectical behavior therapy (DBT), as fashioned by Dr. Marsha Linehan, a psychologist who has diagnosed herself as having borderline personality disorder, for which DBT is an evidence-based treatment.

Mindfulness is yet another Eastern contribution to changing our consciousness in ways that do not carry the consequences and costs of psychoactive drug use and abuse.

PSYCHEDELIC DRUGS (HALLUCINOGENS)

Steve Jobs once said, "Taking LSD was a profound experience, one of the most important things in my life. LSD shows you that there's another side to the coin, and you can't remember it when it wears off, but you know it. It reinforced my sense of what was important—creating great things instead of making money, putting things back into the stream of history and of human consciousness as much as I could."

Psychedelic drugs profoundly alter our consciousness by changing what we see and feel, how we experience ourselves and the world. They can instill a state of being at one with the universe. They have captured human imagination for a long time, well before the sixties, when I came upon them.

Psychedelic agents, such as psilocybin, LSD, and ayahuasca, can produce a sense of wonder that we often leave behind in childhood. It may seem ironic that I list psychedelic drugs as one alternative to psychoactive drugs in pursuing changing our consciousness. However, counterintuitively, new research shows that we must consider their potential utility in strategies to combat the drug epidemic and as paths for research into other psychoactive interventions. They represent yet another alternative that may be more successful, for some, than our otherwise failed efforts.

The Centre for Neuropsychopharmacology at the Imperial College in London has published a study of twenty healthy volunteers who received intravenous LSD on one occasion and a placebo on a second. The pharmaceutical-quality LSD produced "robust psychological effects"—as we would imagine—not just right away but, notably, for some time after the drug was taken. Researchers reported increased optimism and openness two full weeks after taking LSD. While the acute effects at the time the drug was administered included psychotic thinking (e.g., paranoia and delusions), these did not persist, and curiously the subjects did not report distress but rather were apt to describe a positive mood and even a "blissful" experience.

LSD exerts its neurochemical effects on our brain's serotonin system. One particular serotonin receptor, 2A, seems to be central to its effects; when it is blocked by an antagonist specific to this receptor, then the psychedelic effects are not achieved. (This was shown not with LSD but with psilocybin, another psychedelic drug that amplifies serotonin action in the brain.)

The London researchers excluded subjects under twenty-one and those with personal or family histories of mental or substance use disorders or with a significant general medical condition or who were pregnant. But that does not exclude a lot of people who might consider taking LSD.

The London researchers are not new to the science of psychedelics or the seeking of routes to change our reality in beneficial ways. Their work identifies altered connectivity between two regions in the brain, the hippocampus and cortex, strongly correlated with states of "ego-dissolution" and "altered meaning." (The use of microdoses of LSD will be discussed in chapter 6, "Principles of Treatment.")

But LSD isn't the only mind-altering agent with potential medical uses. Psilocybin, or "magic mushrooms," has also been well studied. It has been used at Johns Hopkins and New York University, as well as by the Imperial College, for the treatment of anxiety in cancer patients, and researchers at UCLA have also done pilot work using psilocybin for smoking addiction. Over five hundred administrations of psilocybin at Hopkins and

NYU have not produced any serious negative side effects. Some researchers even wonder about its beneficial effects on addictions other than smoking, as well as its utility in treating people with clinical depression.

Ketamine, which has long been approved by the FDA as an anesthetic for surgery, has also received considerable media (and professional) attention for its rapid treatment of resistant depression. Ketamine has additionally been shown to have prompt effects in diminishing the symptoms of obsessive-compulsive disorder (OCD), a serious, emotionally painful, and functionally impairing condition. Perhaps more research will reveal a role for it for addiction. So far, however, the utility of this drug is limited by its duration, which is usually only one week. Ketamine does not act through the serotonin system; instead, its action is at the glutamate receptor (seldom discussed despite its ubiquity in the brain). However, ketamine is also popular as a club drug, often called Special K, because of its euphoric effects, raising concerns about its abuse, diversion, and potential for addiction.

I am certainly not recommending finding a local drug dealer or knocking on the door of your neighborhood university brain researcher to get some LSD, psilocybin, or ketamine. But like many others, I am hoping that what we learn from these drugs might open new pathways to treat some disabling mental conditions; enable some of us to quiet our fears when ill with cancer or close to passing; and help others who are determined, legal sanctions notwithstanding, to alter their consciousness or to add a touch more creativity and flexibility to their individual and collective worlds.

SOME OLD-FASHIONED APPROACHES

Dr. Harvey Milkman, my great friend of over fifty years and an internationally active expert on addictions, likes to talk about the "meaningful engagement of talents."

He writes, "Engaging one's talents such as playing a favorite sport, sketching a waterfall, hip hop dancing, playing music, or campaigning for a politician you believe in—especially if the activities are perceived as meaningful—is likely to charge up the reward cascade. Through meaningful engagement of talents, we can orchestrate the natural release of serotonin, endorphins, and dopamine, thereby reducing our reliance on alcohol, drugs, or other false props to improve mental and physical well-being."

With his colleague Dr. Kenneth Wanberg, Dr. Milkman notes that we humans derive pleasure by four principal means, or activities. These are physical expression, self-focus, aesthetic discovery, and collective harmony. Physical expression includes exercise and sports (described earlier in this chapter), as well as natural challenges such as wilderness, mountain, and sea adventures. Self-focus includes our attention to our well-being, inner experiences, and calm. Aesthetic discovery includes artistic expression in music, dance, art, theater, writing, painting, photography, and so on, as well as the wonders of nature. Collective harmony, as they describe it, combines the exercise of our minds, intimacy with others, spiritual involvement, and altruism. These four are not mutually exclusive and all build on one another.

I like to think of the "meaningful engagement of talents" as what happens to all of us when we become engrossed in life, relationships, work, and play. Time passes quickly, everyday pains and bothers fade away, boredom evaporates, and our mind is transported in pleasurable ways. What I have described here are some anodynes, effective alternatives, and means of countering the mental malaise and emptiness that can create the conditions for the use and abuse of substances.

Alternatives to substance use and dependence are highly available, diverse, and needed by all of us. They are not mere distractions. They are means by which our lives can be enriched, pain lessened, and pleasure increased. They serve as critical protections against the otherwise destructive use of substances to try to achieve those same ends.

6

PRINCIPLES OF TREATMENT

Doctors are men who prescribe medicines of which they know little, to cure diseases of which they know less, in human beings of whom they know nothing.

—VOLTAIRE

Now the trumpet summons us again—not as a call to bear arms, though arms we need—not as a call to battle, though embattled we are—but a call to bear the burden of a long twilight struggle, year in and year out, "rejoicing in hope, patient in tribulation"—a struggle against the common enemies of man: tyranny, poverty, disease, and war itself.

—JOHN FITZGERALD KENNEDY, INAUGURAL ADDRESS

PART I:
PERSPECTIVES AND PRINCIPLES

Perspective: Neuroscience You
Need to Know and Can Understand

Have you wondered how a (good) clinician, psychiatrist, addiction expert, psychologist, social worker, or independently licensed nurse comes up with his or her recommendations for treatment? What is the critical thinking underlying these recommendations?

As an example, let's look at a comprehensive treatment plan for drug and alcohol addiction—or, more properly, for what is now termed a substance use disorder (SUD). An SUD is characterized as the overuse or dependence on a drug with adverse effects on that person's physical and mental health, as well as negative consequences on others. The use of the substance, whether it is cocaine, OxyContin, heroin, alcohol, marijuana, or any other drug, persists despite clear and serious problems with family, work, and personal relationships. Legal problems also tend to accrue.

Two related fields of science, biological and cognitive neuroscience, have substantially informed the treatment of an SUD, which includes the use of both legal and illicit drugs. Our understanding of the brain, still the most complex organ and system we know of, has grown vastly in recent decades. We have come to understand far better the various parts of our brains, their respective functions, and their neurochemistry and circuitry, as well as how to impact them. We are far from claiming mastery of the central nervous system, but that need not keep us from acting on what we know. Knowledge is what a good doctor or clinician brings to a clinical encounter with a patient and should inform and provide confidence to a patient and family when seeking help. Working together, doctor, patient, and family are what make for the best chance of a successful treatment.

As an example, let's consider a person dependent upon heroin or a prescription analgesic (such as OxyContin, Percodan, or Vicodin), now well recognized as an epidemic in the United States and other countries. The mainstay of SUD treatment has traditionally been 12-step programs such as AA and NA, but today these should only represent but one of a number of interventions that can make a critical difference. That's where neuroscience comes in. Your doctor or other medical or behavioral health professional can, and should, offer more than AA or NA alone. A well-trained clinician can now consider the underlying brain mechanisms driving the addiction and its self-destructive behaviors.

With an understanding of how the brain works when depen-dent on a drug, an informed clinician can develop a comprehen-sive treatment plan for a person with a substance use disorder.

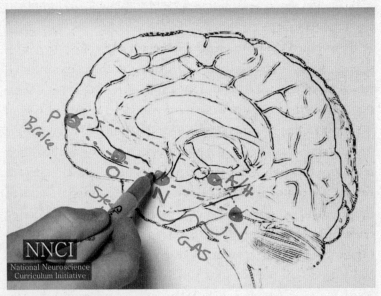

The reward circuit within the brain, shown here with important regions marked, can powerfully influence addiction.

Scientists and mental health clinicians understand that our brains have a reward circuit that powerfully drives our behav-iors. We can use this knowledge to build a treatment plan and to explain to a patient and a family, not just to a fellow clinician or neuroscientist, how to think about and treat addictions.

The two sections of the brain marked *V* and *N* above, for the "ventral tegmental area" and the "nucleus accumbens," are instru-mental to our experience of pleasure (which is necessary for the survival of the species—because pleasures, rewards, also include food, attachment, and sex). When the nerve cells in these areas receive a spike of dopamine, this is like an accelerator pedal. With addiction, that spike is from a drug, not everyday life, hence the idea of an addiction's hijacking our brain from its normal sources of pleasure or reward. (The term *hijack* for how addiction disrupts the brain has been promulgated by the director of the National Institute on Drug Abuse [NIDA], Dr. Nora Volkow.)

Addiction also hijacks the brain in another notable way. Once dependent on a drug, people principally pursue the drug to relieve the misery of withdrawal. This has been called a *negative* (rather than a *positive*) *reinforcer* of behavior. (That is, an action taken to stop feeling bad.) Thus, people with an addiction have a hijacked brain in two ways: they seek both pleasure *and* relief from the discomforts of withdrawal, which are a powerful duo to contend with and try to manage.

Let's return to the brain circuitry we are discussing. Another section, marked *O*, for the "orbital frontal cortex," serves to generate human drive and motivation. This region is also pumped up by the dopamine spike and gets us going, namely, wanting more of what makes us feel good or less of what makes us feel bad. It drives us humans (and animals) to repeat experiences, even if that means swallowing a handful of pain pills or sticking a needle in our arm.

But we humans have evolved past many animals. We now have brains with a highly developed cortex, especially the frontal region (*P*), where our reasoning and judgment reside. The "prefrontal cortex" can control our drives, put some brakes on the accelerator pedal when going at a high RPM, so to speak.

Finally, there are the *A/H*, for the "amygdala" and "hippocampus," which are regions of the brain that store memories of what we find rewarding. They also register what is salient to the reward, namely the cues associated with its source. Remember that Pavlov's dogs salivated, over time, to the bell, not to the food; that mental change is known as a conditioned response. While it is the reward that drives us to repeat a behavior, to survive or simply to enjoy life, it is the cues that get us going *and* offer important opportunities for intervention.

In a brain addicted to drugs, this five-region circuit becomes pirated away (hijacked) because the opioid (heroin or analgesic pain pills, for example) directly boosts dopamine in the *V* and *N* sections of the brain. This spike then triggers the circuit to powerfully fire, which drives a person to repetitively seek sources of the pleasure. However, in this case the aim is not love, food, or altruism; it is securing more substances of abuse.

A doctor or clinician today has ways to construct a comprehensive treatment plan that targets the various components of the circuit and thereby increase a person's likelihood of successful recovery. Each intervention is additive, and their sum is useful, often essential, given the power of an addiction. With problems of this magnitude we know that the more we arm our brains with, the better we will do. Several examples:

- A number of medications are now available, and their use is called *medication-assisted treatment of addiction,* or *MAT.* They can, for example, block the effect of the drug in the *V* and *N* regions of the brain. More about these later in this chapter.
- Motivation to resist desire to reexperience the spike in the *O* region can be enhanced by *motivational interviewing (MI),* a brief technique that has for many years been used with people with addictions and is now popular in helping individuals with any number of problem behaviors (e.g., overeating, tobacco use, and gambling).
- The section of our brain that helps us use good judgment,

the *P* region, can be substantially assisted by a variety of interventions, including NA/AA, family psychoeducation and
support, and promoting coping skills, such as surrounding
yourself with people who are not using or abusing substances,
eating and sleeping well, and stress-reduction practices such
as yoga and slow breathing.
* Finally, the *A/H* regions can also be positively impacted,
especially the *H* region. Environmental triggers can drive
cravings and relapse; these include the sight of a needle or
a pill, contact with people using or dealers, commercials
about pain relief, even reports of the overdose deaths of
Philip Seymour Hoffman or Prince. *Cognitive behavioral
therapy (CBT)* can help a person with a substance use disorder to avoid or have a reduced response to a trigger.

A comprehensive plan for a person with a drug addiction could,
therefore—hopefully kindled by motivational interviewing—offer
the patient, and supportive loved ones, a solution potentially
including medication-assisted treatment, 12-step recovery, family
psychoeducation, CBT, and a number of wellness activities such
as yoga and yogic breathing, meditation, mindfulness, exercise,
and a nutritional diet, as well as the company of those dedicated
to life, not addiction. This is more than a menu of services: it
is an essential compilation of what can save a life and promote
recovery.

If I, or a loved one, had an addiction, I would want a clinician or clinical team who thought this way. Can an argument be
made against comprehensive treatment of this sort? Not that I
know of. But it does require informed professionals who recognize the power of attacking tough problems in a variety of ways
that augment one another, and who talk with, engage, and help

patients to help themselves. That also means that an informed patient, family, and public should expect no less.

Michael Wildman was admitted to McLean Hospital, where I was medical director, after countless unsuccessful efforts to get his substance use under control. He was in his forties, handsome, with great charm. But his family, who still stood by him, were running out of patience and were convinced he was going to hurt himself or someone else as a result of his carelessness and impulsivity.

I had arranged for admission, and he was flown on a private plane from where he was hospitalized in another state. On board, the security people asked to accompany him somehow thought he would be less trouble if he had his way with the liquor cabinet. Michael liked to drink, could down a liter of vodka in short order, and liked to mix the vodka with stimulants such as cocaine or tranquilizers such as Valium when they were available. When I met him at the admissions department, he was intoxicated and insulting to the staff. He was a little less obnoxious with me, I think because he knew I was the source of the detox meds he wanted, which would ease his withdrawal.

I put him on a detoxification regimen of Librium, folic acid, lots of fluids, and nutritional supplements. We monitored his vital signs (blood pressure, pulse, respiration, and temperature), and he had an uneventful withdrawal. But then what? What might make a difference this time, unlike the many times he had tried before?

With colleagues at the hospital, I set up a program of individual (with me) and group counseling, which included relapse prevention and CBT; daily exercise in whatever form he wanted, though usually he wanted none; training in meditation focused on his breath; and regular meetings with his family, his biggest supporters even as he caused them immense pain. He began and sustained attendance at daily AA and sometimes NA meetings. We weaned him, if you will, not only from intoxicants but from red meat, french fries, sugary beverages, and sweets, and he came to like a Mediterranean diet rich in fish and vegetables.

When it was time for him to leave the hospital, we knew his risk of relapse would be high. He entered first a sober home, then "graduated" to his own apartment not far from the hospital and its outpatient services, including me. His mother came and stayed with him initially, which he did not like, but soon he was on his own and building a life in recovery, which included going back to work.

We did not rely on AA/NA alone, or counseling alone, or just family meetings. We helped him learn the mind-body technique of breathing, how to eat well, and to try to walk every day to have a physically healthy heart. The new, nondrinking relationships, improved family relations, and employment—all that built up his heart in other ways. Comprehensive treatment is what he received, and it worked. That's what we are talking about for everyone facing the ravages of addiction.

Principles of Good Addiction Treatment

In my book for families, I wrote about a set of principles for good mental health care that are no different for the addictions. They are as follows.

- Screening for illnesses to be treated should be standard practice in primary care and schools, with early intervention when problems are detected.

- Treatment should be comprehensive and continuous.
- Treatment should be evidence based or evidence informed.
  - All treatment should be measurement based, aimed at measurable goals, monitored, and used to continuously improve care.
- Treatment should be safe.
- Treatment should be collaborative.
  - Treatment should include "shared decision making."
  - Treatment should account for patient preferences.
  - Collaboration should extend, whenever possible, to families and friends.
- *Similia similibus curantur* (like cures like) and *spiritus contra spiritum* (spirits—alcohol—depraves/destroys our spiritual thirst).
- Treatment should meet linguistic and cultural needs.
- Treatment should be recovery oriented.

The essential principle of prevention has its own earlier chapter. Screening has also been addressed in that chapter.

Before we look at these principles, let's look at how humans change. No book on human behavior, especially on the addictions, is complete without reference to what has been termed *the stages of change*.

Starting in the late 1970s, and culminating in their breakthrough book in 1984 known among professionals as *The Stages of Change*, James O. Prochaska and Carlo DiClemente developed and revealed a model of change that was agnostic to the many schools of psychotherapy that had emerged in the last century.

Instead, using the prevalent therapies as a platform, they identified six stages by which we humans change.

The six stages are precontemplation (not ready); contemplation (getting ready); preparation (within a month of taking action); action; maintenance; and, finally, termination (confident there will be no relapse).

Talking with somebody about taking action—for example, setting a date to quit smoking or reduce alcohol consumption—who is in the precontemplation phase not only does not work, it can drive them further from taking later action. While these stages can be fluid, they are important for clinicians, family and friends, and policy makers to understand so they can fashion interventions accordingly.

On to the principles for good mental health treatment, all equally applicable for the treatment of addiction.

Treatment Should Be Comprehensive and Continuous

The neuroscience section above illustrates how comprehensive care is considered and implemented. Addictive disorders have complex drivers and benefit from intervening at as many places in the human brain, mind, and behavior as possible. This is one area where doing less is certainly less.

Continuous care means that treatment does not start and stop for any reason or as a result of reluctance or difficulties in obtaining care. Individual reluctance and these difficulties are at work most of the time and thus are critical barriers to be overcome. We don't get better from any condition unless we see its treatment through to its natural conclusion. Continuous care does not necessarily mean intensive care forever, but it does mean maintaining a good working relationship with caregivers and staying the course. Clinicians and clinical services need to be welcoming, accessible, respectful, and vigorously attentive to engaging and retaining patients in care.

Treatment Should Be Evidence Based (or Evidence Informed) and to "Target"

A great deal has been learned and disseminated about what works in mental health and addictive treatments. Responsible, professional caregivers are always looking for new information and practices that will close what has been called the science-to-practice gap. The evidence referred to here is what has been studied and replicated by trustworthy researchers (i.e., it is evidence based) or is promising but has yet to appear in medical journals (i.e., it is evidence informed). That is what we should want our clinician to put on the table when we meet to discuss treatment options.

But that is not enough. Treatment to target is crucial. We would not begin a diabetes or hypertension treatment or care for a malignancy without a clear measurement baseline, such as HgA1c (a blood test that determines ongoing sugar control in our body, which is more accurate over time than daily blood-glucose readings), blood pressure, or tumor size and activity, that can be regularly monitored to ensure that the treatment is working or can be altered if it is not. This is called treatment-to-target or measurement-based care.

Screening instruments to identify a condition and to provide data points, measurements, that can be tracked over time are essential to measurement-based care. Our blood pressure, our heart rate, our lipids, our sugars, are all measured to provide data points for medical management. So too can problem behaviors be screened for, measured, and monitored. In people with addictions, the use of quantifiable measures to assess clinical progress is in its infancy, though research work has used measures for some time.

Treatment Should Be Safe

As some know, I am fond of the history of gunshot wounds, which aptly demonstrates *primum non nocere*—first, do no harm.

Back in the fourteenth century, battlefield surgeons abandoned an ancient, safe approach to treating wounds, especially gunshot wounds, and began pouring boiling oil into the open lesions. The earlier practice, dating back to the Egyptians, of gentle wound care by removing debris, carefully washing with water, and covering the wound to allow natural healing was replaced by filling it with boiling oil. This unsafe and disastrous practice persisted for two hundred years, until one day no boiling oil was handy for the surgeons. They resorted to the ancient technique and discovered that gentle, safe care was clearly superior.

This story reminds us that every treatment needs to be as safe and as gentle as possible. Safety in treatment pertains not just to medications but to individual and group therapies, to nutritional approaches to well-being, and to the day-to-day communities of people and the environments in which people with substance-use problems live.

Treatment Should Be Collaborative

This means that care must have at its core the value that patients can be their best advocates and agents and should hence be engaged in what is called shared decision making. Dr. Pat Deegan was an originator of this approach and continues to shape our field. Collaborative care recognizes that all chronic illnesses are best managed when the patient, and family, when possible, are fully engaged as active partners in treatment.

In *Born to Run*, Bruce Springsteen's autobiography, we come upon a second book dedication late in this 510-page personal odyssey, penned by one of the greatest musical spokespersons of our time. Springsteen's father was an alcoholic, prone to violent outbursts. While Springsteen himself has been free of substance-use problems, he has suffered many severe bouts of depression. He writes about his long-term treatment for that disorder in this book.

The Boss (as he is known) tells the reader, "The results of my work with Dr. [Wayne] Myers and my debt to him are at the heart of this book." "Doc" Myers was Springsteen's New York City psychiatrist and therapist from 1983—when the Boss faced "bramble-filled darkness" and a stubborn feeling that there would be no exit—until shortly before Myers died in 2009. In 1983, Springsteen would soon achieve fame and fortune. But these don't make for happiness and are poor anodynes to depression and hopelessness. Springsteen writes that Myers "guided me to the strength and freedom I needed to love things and be loved." For many years Springsteen's treatment worked, but that did not keep him from relapsing into depression when he turned sixty. But he had developed trust and confidence, a sense of how a doctor and patient can work together, found another doctor, and recovered, slowly, over a number of years.

As a psychiatrist, I cannot think of a finer testimonial, unsolicited and authentic, to my field and to those patients (and families) who work to overcome a mental or substance use disorder.

Springsteen's treatment was surely collaborative, and he stands as an example not just of musical greatness but of human frailty, as well as resilience and recovery.

I am reminded, as well, of a patient I treated who at first was evasive and resistant to treatment. A talented financial-services executive in his forties, he was referred to me by a managing partner who witnessed rapidly shifting moods, including irritability; increasing lateness; failure to complete transactions; and covering up for failed responsibilities. The executive had been a great asset to his company, and before they let him go, they wanted to see if they could preserve him.

Samuel Gold, as I will call him, arrived late for our first visit. He was a bit unkempt despite wearing expensive clothing and likely $1,000 shoes. He immediately took control of the meeting by saying he did not want to be there and was only doing so to satisfy his boss. In his view, he had no problems except an overcontrolling manager. I tried to meet him, at first, on neutral ground, asking about where he lived, his family, his work, his friends, his interests. But he was surly, muttering curt answers and saying he was busy and needed to leave.

I said that he could leave anytime he wanted, but he would not leave behind the demand from his firm that he understand his problems, all observable and persistent, and take action toward solving them. Unless that happened, I imagined (and he reluctantly agreed) he would soon be packing up his desk and surrendering his security clearance. That created the basis of an alliance, not quite for treatment, but, because I held the power to prevent his dismissal, the grounds for a kind of partnership.

Once I had his attention, I started to ask what he wanted

for himself and his family. He liked making money but was also a responsible family man and involved in his temple and community, or at least he had been. He grasped that all that was in peril, but not that he had the power to preserve what he wanted and needed.

I learned that he had had two orthopedic surgeries, in rather short order, a couple of years earlier for sports-related shoulder and knee injuries. He had been prescribed Percodan postoperatively for his knee procedure and OxyContin after the shoulder surgery, appropriate for short-term pain relief but generally not for ongoing, nonterminal treatment. He was given a month's supply of medication each time, and he subsequently requested and received refills for the pain that enervated him and interfered with travel and everyday activities at home and work. He said he had no time for physical rehab and that the pills were his way of keeping going. But soon he was on that substance-induced merry-go-round of relief and intoxication followed by withdrawal. His performance began to suffer and he became short with colleagues and at home.

After his orthopedic doctors stopped his supply of opioids, he purchased them on the black market—an addiction he hid from his firm, but that did not escape notice by his wife. I stressed that while what he valued was not yet lost, it was surely in peril, and asked what if anything he wanted to do about it. The first session ended and he agreed to return for another. My job was to enable him to own his problem, not blame others, and to see that he could be helped if he worked at it, had the support of his family, and received good treatment. After a number of meetings, he became ready to quit drugs and recover the life he wanted. My therapeutic opponent had become a partner. At last, he could begin to walk the road of both physical and substance-use recovery. Samuel Gold's is a success story, especially in that he came early to treatment, recognized that he had a lot to lose, had important supports at home and work, and had the resources to support an effective treatment. Not everyone is so blessed, but treatment works—just sometimes not right away.

Related to the value of an authentic partnership between patient and clinician is attention to patient preferences. We all do what we want to, when possible, and our adherence to treatments and self-care is no different. Some people prefer therapy, others medications, some all that is possible. Some value regular appointments, while others prefer a more ad hoc arrangement. Some like phone calls and emails, others to meet in person. When we ask about and respond to patient preferences, we have someone far more likely to get the hard work of treatment done.

An essential corollary is that collaboration extends, whenever possible, to families and friends. No mental health system will ever be able to identify serious behavioral problems as early as a loving family or close friend. They are both the elements of a needed and effective early-warning system as well as the most enduring supports a person can have. They see the trouble, the drift toward relapse, daily. Many times it is they who seek help for their loved one. Families and friends (though, of course, not all of them) are among the strongest allies clinicians will have.

Similia Similibus Curantur and Spiritus Contra Spiritum

Harry Stack Sullivan, MD (1892–1949), was a highly innovative American psychiatrist. His particular interest was in working with people with serious mental illnesses, particularly psychotic conditions such as schizophrenia. He was, as well, one of the first proponents of using people with histories of illness who were in recovery to assist in the treatment of those whose conditions had not yet stabilized or improved. His work exemplified *similia similibus curantur*.

Around the time that Dr. Sullivan was advancing "like cures like," there came along—also in the United States—Alcoholics Anonymous. In Ohio, in 1935, two severe alcoholics, Bill W., a New York stockbroker, and Dr. Bob S., an Akron surgeon, met and began what has become a lasting fellowship across the world. Fundamental to AA is not just its spiritual element but that others suffering from the same condition are integral to recovery.

As the story goes, Bill W. had sought help from a friend, "Roland H.," who had consulted with the legendary Swiss psychiatrist Carl Jung. So began the theme of spirituality in AA. Jung emphasized the necessity of spirituality as a powerful foil against alcohol (spirits).

Jung is even mentioned in AA's *Big Book*. When Roland H. asked Jung if there was any way for a chronic alcoholic to fully recover, Jung reportedly replied:

Yes, there is. Exceptions to cases such as yours have been occurring since early times. Here and there, once in a while, alcoholics have had what are called vital spiritual experiences. To me these are phenomena. They appear to be in the nature of huge emotional displacements and rearrangements. Ideas, emotions, and attitudes which were once the guiding forces of the lives of these men are suddenly cast to one side, and a completely new set of conceptions and motives begin to dominate them. In fact, I have been trying to produce some such emotional rearrangement within you. With many individuals the methods which I employed are successful, but I have never been successful with an alcoholic of your description.

A record exists of a letter Dr. Jung sent to Bill W., many years later, emphasizing the transformative power of the spirit and, as well, of human connectedness, both of which gave rise to AA and its development. Part of the letter is reproduced below:

Dear Mr. Wilson,

[Roland H.'s] craving for alcohol was the equivalent on a low level of the spiritual thirst of our being for wholeness, expressed in medieval language: the union with God. . . .

The only right and legitimate way to such an experience is that it happens to you in reality—and it can only happen to you when you walk on a path, which leads you to higher understanding. You might be led to that goal by an act of grace or through a personal and honest contact with friends, or through a higher education of the mind beyond the confines of mere rationalism. . . .

You see, Alcohol in Latin is "spiritus" and you use the same word for the highest religious experience as well as for the most depraving poison. The helpful formula therefore is spiritus contra spiritum.

Thanking you again for your kind letter

    I remain

        yours sincerely

        Carl Jung

In AA, NA, or one of the other 12-step programs that grew up around them, a core principle of addiction care for many is active engagement in a community of other recovering individuals. For many people, spirituality is an internal and necessary experience, and fellowship with others who are addicts is mutative—just as it was for Bill W., Dr. Bob, and Roland H. Families have also become part of this movement, for example with Al-Anon, a group designed for family members and friends of people with addictions, who are often the first to see signs of relapse and can be the most important and enduring sources of support for a person in recovery.

Treatment Should Meet
Linguistic and Cultural Needs

We hear this all the time: Unless clinicians understand the beliefs, values, history, and language of those they treat, how can they succeed? This principle, however, needs to lean into the concept *let not the perfect be the enemy of the good.*

The use of translators, interpreters, is one way to bridge the gap, as is having nonprofessional workers native to their communities assist in treating people with all chronic diseases, including the addictions. Asking what people think, prefer, and value goes a long way, as well, to helping those who have a different background than we do.

Dr. Roberto Lewis-Fernández, MD, MPH, and his colleagues have developed useful approaches to cultural competence that can be adopted broadly and successfully.

Cultural competence in health care, including mental health and the addictions, seeks to understand people's experiences with their lives and their illnesses. What patients know and value informs a clinician's approach to them, and in addition, people's backgrounds, lived experiences, and communities can become important guides in helping them take greater control over their health and well-being. Finally, family and friends are recognized and included whenever possible.

While language is important, these other elements of a culturally informed approach to clinical care are even more essential.

Treatment Should Be Recovery Oriented

The essence of this principle is that clinician and patient share the view that the treatment aims toward a clean and sober life (or as close as possible) and toward the reduction of the emotional problems that helped create and sustain substance use. *Those are essential, but not enough.* Recovery-oriented treatment also has as its goal that people rebuild their lives and recover relationships, functioning, contribution, and purpose. Patients and families need to seek and stay with clinicians and programs that are recovery oriented.

Other Aspects of Our Lives

Our behaviors, our habits—such as excessive and poor eating, more than moderate drinking, smoking, physical inactivity and poor sleep, sugary beverages, high-salt and processed-food intake—drive the lion's share (40 percent!) of ill health and early demise. Another 30 percent of our health appears attributable to our genes. But we now recognize, through the science of epigenetics, that DNA is turned on or off by its exposure to our environment and what we do and don't do. If we are to be healthier and live longer, we must look beyond hospitals, doctors, and clinics because together they account for only 10 percent of our health. This was put brilliantly by Professor Paula Lantz when she wrote that Americans are prone to "mistaking health care for health."

Impact of Different Factors on Risk of Premature Death

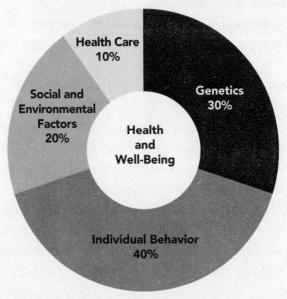

SOURCE: Schroeder, SA. (2007). "We Can Do Better—Improving the Health of the American People," *NEIM.* 357:1221–28.

Poor health and premature death are determined by a number of factors, with individual behavior as a major driver.

We also must always keep hope alive. People with substance use disorders can and do recover. That takes good treatment, hard work, time, ongoing support, and belief in the possibility of recovery. People with addictions can get on the path to recovery—but it is hard to predict when that will happen. Some will stop or control use on their own. For some of those who seek treatment, it will be early, even after one or two rehabilitation programs. For others it may take five, ten, or twenty rehab programs, and the pain and suffering of too many relapses. Their loved ones and clinical providers need to sustain hope that recovery can happen during what can be protracted and dark times.

The darkest moments, the most deadly, are when hope evaporates, which is when exile from family, friends, and communities, as well as suicide, are most likely.

After the movie screening, Chris Herren settled onto a stool, microphone in hand, for the Q and A and rubbed his left knee—the knee that hurt too much to continue to play for the Boston Celtics and accelerated his dependence on drugs and alcohol.

The occasion was a preview of an ESPN documentary on the life of this gifted athlete from Fall River, Massachusetts, who wowed them at Durfee High School and in a pro career that was as brilliant and transient as a comet in the autumn sky.

This basketball guard displayed incredible moves from his days on the playgrounds of Fall River, to Boston College, to Fresno State under the wing of the legendary coach Jerry Tarkanian. Drafted by the Denver Nuggets in 1999, he was traded to the Boston Celtics in 2000. Man, could this handsome, beaming, arm-pumping athlete drive, pass, and shoot. Even under the influence.

But ultimately, his arms were where he stuck a needle loaded with heroin. He traded a shelf of trophies for a rap sheet of felony convictions. His fans booed him. His family cried from the pain he brought upon himself and them. He converted "nothing but net" into nothing but a life compulsively driven by dope. As painful as that is to watch, imagine what it must have been to live.

Chris Herren went from drinking and marijuana to his first line of cocaine when he was eighteen. But it was opioid pain pills that took him to the major leagues of drug addiction. First it was Percodan, then Vicodin, but not until OxyContin did he become a pro. Life centered no longer on basketball: it centered on scoring a pill that has become a nationwide killer of people, not just pain.

Herren continued taking OxyContin not to get high, but to manage the withdrawal, the "dope sickness" that comes when the body is denied a substance upon which it has become dependent. When his wife took his car keys so he couldn't drive to his drug dealer twelve miles away, he got on his ten-speed bicycle and pedaled, on the highway, to get his fix. When he went to play basketball abroad—no longer US material—first in Italy, then China, Turkey, even Iran, he upped his game to heroin when pills were not readily available.

He had been to rehab a few times, in college and the pros. I have learned no one ever knows when the lifelong process of recovery will "take"—when the repetitive relapses will transform into days, weeks, months, and years of sobriety. For people with addiction, families, and my fellow clinicians, the message is *never give up*. We may not be able to predict when it will happen, but it does, more often than we imagine.

Just as it happened with Chris Herren. He was blessed with a loving and enduringly supportive family. He had not only the gift of being a great ballplayer, but he had (has) the gift of being amiable—the kind of person you want to succeed, almost no matter how much he has hurt you and others. He received good treatment and used it. It was Daytop, a drug-treatment program in the New York area, founded in the 1960s, and the unbending demands of its counselors, that helped Herren find his heart and soul once again. The man has emerged from the drug.

Chris Herren is the father of three children and still married to his childhood sweetheart. He is now years into his sobriety and coaching youth basketball. His smile warms your heart. You want him to win. He tells his story with humility and with the hope that someone, some youth or aging person with an addiction, or person at risk for a life too full of ruin, will find hope, treatment, and the road to recovery. One day at a time.

PART II:
TREATMENT

In this section, I will present a variety of treatments available (or promising) for people with substance use disorders and their families. I do not aim, as noted in earlier chapters, to be encyclopedic in this discussion. Instead, my goal is to point out that many diverse approaches exist, that generally they are complementary and additive, and that patients and families need to find their own best solutions.

But before we get to those solutions I want to touch on two matters. The first is a cautionary note because of the desperation that addictions can produce in substance users and their families. The second is the vital importance of detecting and treating *both* co-occurring mental disorders, including depression, PTSD, bipolar and schizophrenic illnesses, and borderline personality, *and* co-occurring physical problems, especially chronic pain. No one is apt to get better from an addiction unless mental and physical problems are properly diagnosed and managed, and vice versa.

Beware the Hucksters

Results guaranteed! 92% recover! Pool, personal chef, and equine therapy included!

A promotion for snake oil? For a destination resort? Not exactly. That's what families might read when they go online, desperate and frightened that a loved one with an addiction may die unless he or she is treated and gets better. That's what those in the throes of an addiction read as well, and the seduction can be alluring.

The addiction-treatment "industry," not including public, state, city, and county treatment programs, is principally for-profit—and it is big business. Private not-for-profits are in the business as well, with their CEOs and medical directors making high-six-figure incomes. Annually, industry revenues are estimated to be $34 billion (2013), as we see in a screenshot and voice-over in the riveting documentary *The Business of Recovery*, released in 2015. Addiction is ubiquitous in our society, and its toll is grave.

If the mental health–care system is troubled, and it surely is, the substance use treatment system is even more so—but it has largely escaped notice. That leaves patients and their families all the more subject to its false claims, inadequate treatments, and financial exploitation.

One great overstatement the addiction-treatment industry propagates is that the 12-step method of recovery is extraordinarily effective. "Ninety percent of recovery centers are based on AA," the documentary I mentioned above tells us as we virtually visit some of the best-known and most (financially) successful programs in this country. AA means the 12 steps, a spiritual approach to recovery, developed by Dr. Bob and Bill W., as described earlier. Studies of AA estimate that it works for 5–10 percent of those who use it. One in twenty, maybe one in ten, respond to AA, yet *90 percent* of the treatment programs, including the most preeminent (not to mention the most expensive), are based on and adhere, often principally, to a method with a low response rate.

Beware the hucksters. Prospective patients and families are *not* apt to be told how small the chances of response are before entering what may be a monochromatic treatment program (however fine the amenities may be) and beginning to pay tens or scores of thousands of dollars every month. Some patients and families spend vast sums of money for treatment and have mortgaged their homes or spent their savings or money meant for the education of other children. Too many addiction-program directors, in all earnestness, swear by AA as if it works a lot better than it does.

The burden, caveat emptor (buyer beware), will generally be on prospective consumers of services to ask what the treatment program includes before they enroll. If they don't hear about a comprehensive approach, if they are *only* sung the AA tune, I'd recommend they keep their credit card in their pocket.

I do not mean to disparage AA, NA, and their related 12-step programs. These can and have helped countless people. They are accessible, free, and anonymous. But beware of programs that rely only on this approach. There is more to be had—and other offerings will only increase the chances of recovery.

Co-occurring Disorders

How can people manage the complex challenges of addiction if they are also clinically depressed, unable to mobilize or care, or, worse, think they would be better off dead? Or if they are, instead, living a life with manic and depressive swings, paranoid delusions, and persecutory hallucinations, seen with psychotic illnesses? Or if they suffer from the ongoing mental and physical depletion brought on by emotional trauma, including PTSD?

How can people manage the complex challenges of addiction if they have blood sugars bouncing around from uncontrolled diabetes, or chest pain from walking up a flight of stairs, or difficulty breathing, or knees or hips burning up with the inflammation and pain of arthritis?

Of course, these questions answer themselves. Yet so many people with substance use disorders do not have their co-occurring mental or physical condition identified, accurately diagnosed, and effectively treated. The price they pay—and that we pay too in their high use of medical and social services—is great in human suffering, family disruption and stress, and the draining of personal and governmental treasuries.

Many inroads are being made to ensure the detection and treatment of co-occurring conditions, especially in primary medical care, specialty mental health and substance use disorder programs, enlightened business settings, employee-assistance programs, and community-based organizations. People with substance use disorders and their loved ones should be sure that the identification and treatment of any active mental or medical problems are at the top of their to-do list if they want to enhance the chances of success.

Former congressman Patrick J. Kennedy's story shows us the importance of identifying and treating a co-occurring mental illness. In 1995, at the age of twenty-seven, Mr. Kennedy became the youngest member of the Congress of the United States, having been elected to the House of Representatives from his home state of Rhode Island. When he left Congress in 2011, a more-than-sixty-year era of a Kennedy serving in Washington ended. (Patrick Kennedy is the son of the famed former US senator Ted Kennedy and the nephew of former president John F. Kennedy and former attorney general Bobby Kennedy.)

Patrick Kennedy has been unsparing in his revelations about himself, dating back to his teenage years. He reports having had depressive, anxiety, and manic symptoms and that he has been diagnosed with bipolar (manic-depressive) disorder. His heavy use of alcohol, mixed with cocaine and for many years opioid pain pills such as OxyContin and Percodan, was persistent and put him on a path to destruction of all he valued.

But not until his bipolar illness was detected and treated did he gain control, hard-won, over his substance use disorder. But he did. Today, Patrick Kennedy has over six years of sobriety.

Treatment

Not every treatment works for every type of substance use (or behavioral) disorder, and individual responses vary considerably. Remember set and setting from chapter 1? The combination of what happens inside us, biologically and psychologically, and the profound influences of our respective circumstances call for flexibility and persistence in finding the right combination of recovery actions for each individual. These actions must also be specific to the present moment in the condition.

Below we will briefly look at a number of interventions, chosen because of their diversity and both their research and empirical evidence. This will have its limits as a compilation because I am not covering tobacco—the greatest cause of preventable morbidity and mortality, and hence a book in itself—or providing a list of every known treatment for every known substance of abuse. As in other parts of this book, I seek to give the reader illustrations and perspective. Those are my reasons for any omissions the reader may discover.

Spirituality

A fundamental approach to addictions is through spirituality, with or without a formal institutional religion.

It is hard not to think of Marx's comment that "religion is the opiate of the masses." His meaning, I believe, was disdainful. By spirituality I mean that which is or becomes sacred to an individual, which does not necessarily include adherence to a religious institution with its particular beliefs, doctrines, and worship practices. I believe we all hunger for lives of meaning and purpose, and an inner, buoying sense of connection to others, not a life of isolation. Spirituality can provide for those fundamental needs.

The English word *spirit* derives from the Latin *spiritus*, which connotes breath and aspiration, meaning taking in air, or, less literally, a life force. Spirituality does not preclude a belief in science or rationality, as we see among so many great scientists and thinkers who appreciate and honor our human place in an incomprehensible and awesome universe—those who are deeply alert to the beauty, wonder, and mystery of nature and life.

Spirituality, sometimes voiced as faith, is protective against alcoholism and drug abuse. Those who hold to a spiritual existence, who sense a more universal "power" than that possessed by humans, are less likely to develop an addiction. Holding to spiritual beliefs, to faith in its secular meaning, is instrumental to recovery from a host of traumas and conditions, including addictions. In my work overseeing the mental health response to a number of major human-made and natural disasters (such as 9/11 and Hurricane Sandy), I learned that having faith was a predictor of mastering the trauma and rebuilding a life. No surprise, then, that spirituality or faith would serve individuals whose lives have been ravaged by addiction. AA makes that plain. People who have developed a spiritual dimension to their lives are better able to achieve *and* sustain sobriety.

12-Step Recovery

The *Big Book* of AA prescribes its twelve steps, which are the path a person with an addiction must follow to recover and rebuild a life.

The Twelve Steps

1. We admitted we were powerless over alcohol and that our lives had become unmanageable.
2. Came to believe that a power greater than ourselves could restore us to sanity.
3. Made a decision to turn our will and our lives over to the care of God, as we understood Him.
4. Made a searching and fearless moral inventory of ourselves.
5. Admitted to God, to ourselves, and to another human being the exact nature of our wrongs.
6. Were entirely ready to have God remove all these defects of character.
7. Humbly asked Him to remove our shortcomings.
8. Made a list of all persons we had harmed and became willing to make amends to them all.
9. Made direct amends to such people, whenever possible, except when to do so would injure them or others.
10. Continued to take personal inventory and when wrong promptly admitted it.
11. Sought through prayer and meditation to improve our conscious contact with God, as we understood Him, praying only for knowledge of His will for us and the power to carry it out.
12. Having had a spiritual awakening as the result of these steps, we tried to carry this message to alcoholics and to practice these principles in all our affairs.

Twelve-step programs are typified by AA, NA, and related groups for families and teenagers. They are offered for a variety of specific drugs, including alcohol, opioids, cocaine, nicotine, and marijuana, and for behavioral addictions such as gambling, sex, and food. Those who work the program are expected to progress through the twelve steps.

Remarkably, AA and its sibling services exist without any central organization or any external financial contributions. Anonymity is fundamental to meetings and participation. But a person in need can find a meeting almost anywhere, almost every day, as well as a sponsor, a person of the same gender who, usually, has a minimum of one year of sobriety, has been through the twelve steps, and is available to help a newly sober (or striving to be sober) person through the steps.

Some balk at the explicit spirituality in the twelve steps, especially when it is regarded as synonymous with religion. But, again, it is not: religions are based on institutions with specific beliefs and practices, whereas spirituality is individualistic and can take many forms.

As a component of a comprehensive treatment, a 12-step program can be useful. Meetings are also highly accessible, available 24-7, and free.

SMART

SMART (Self-Management and Recovery Training) is an alternative to AA that seeks to enable participants to take control of their problems instead of regarding themselves as being powerless, as 12-step programs assert.

Participants are offered a "4-Point Program [that] offers tools and techniques":

1. Building and maintaining motivation
2. Coping with urges
3. Managing thoughts, feelings, and behaviors
4. Living a balanced life

Unlike AA, which everyone seems to know about, SMART is not well-known, which is unfortunate. It can be a desirable alternative to a spiritual approach to recovery from substances, while also being highly useful, accessible, and free.

Motivational Interviewing (MI) or Motivational Enhancement (ME)

If any of the interventions offered here meet the standard of universality, this one does.

Motivational interviewing is nonjudgmental. There are no moralistic judgments about a person or his or her behaviors. Nor does it allow a person to self-flagellate with negative, abusive comments. Quite the opposite: MI starts by recognizing that an individual is doing something for powerful reasons. MI is a cognitive technique to help people overcome their internal ambivalence to change, to appreciate they will gain more than they will lose by changing a habit; with MI, changes first occur internally before they appear in behavior. MI also appreciates that letting go means losing something, and none of us tolerates loss well.

But we can better bear change when we know that something we want lies ahead. That something may be looking good for a wedding or a reunion, not spending $150 a week on marijuana or alcohol, and not having to sneak around to have a smoke. What matters is not what the doctor wants, but what the patient wants to achieve. Every (small) step is important. Behaving differently is incremental. And we all need ongoing support from people who understand it is hard to let go of what has served our needs. The following example may illustrate the effectiveness of MI.

A young mother goes to her pediatrician with her son, who is experiencing repeated ear infections. The physician notes that smoke exposure (through secondhand smoke) is a significant factor for children who have ear infections. The mother, indeed, is a smoker. Her doctor "counsels" the mother in a confrontational and blaming way. The mother can't wait to get out of the doctor's office and is not at all likely to change her smoking habits. This is not MI; it will drive a patient, any person, away from what they know inside needs to be done.

The same doctor, with the same patient, can offer and receive a very different experience. The doctor can ask open-ended, nonjudgmental questions and reflect back to the patient what she has said. The pediatrician can also enlist her patient in problem solving and ask the patient what she thinks she can do as first steps. The patient is thus engaged, perhaps even relieved to be finally talking about her problem(s), and is far more likely to take some critical first steps in managing her tobacco addiction.

William Miller, PhD, was a pioneer in MI, dating back to the early 1980s. His book with Dr. Stephen Rollnick remains one of the best references we have on this subject. What Miller and Rollnick describe is an interpersonal approach that is truly collaborative, a means to mobilize a person's own motivation to change. Clinicians who employ MI do not fight with patients' natural resistance to change, but rather help the patients see their ambivalence to change while supporting that part of them ready to take a step toward recovery and better self-care. Limited, achievable goals are set, monitored together with the patient, and starts and stops are expected and empathized with—all the while maintaining a belief in the patient's intrinsic strengths. MI began with the treatment of addictive conditions, but its use has spread widely to primary care and the management of chronic health conditions such as hypertension, diabetes, asthma, HIV/AIDS, obesity, and depression.

Whatever may be your background, training, or professional or lay status, this intervention is one to know.

Cognitive Behavioral Therapy (CBT)

How we think affects how we feel and behave. That is the central premise of CBT, which has become widespread in substance use and mental disorder treatments.

Aaron T. Beck, MD, first popularized this creative approach to mental and behavioral problems some decades ago, and it was later extended to addictive disorders.

Imagine a person with an alcohol problem who is in recovery passing a favorite bar or getting a call from an old drinking buddy. That is what we see in *The Man with the Golden Arm*, the film mentioned at the beginning of this book.

The cue is as powerful as the substance itself; after a while—as with Pavlov's dogs, who salivated at the bell, not the food—it becomes a conditioned response. The cue can trigger what Beck and others have called "automatic thoughts," which are often firmly held negative thoughts a person has about himself or herself, such as "I don't deserve to be doing well" or "I am worthless." In response, his or her mood deteriorates and even blood pressure and heart rate can change for the worse. Memories of relief from alcohol, the creeping thought of "Just one drink," come into their minds, and relapse is likely.

CBT is meant to be time limited (eight to twelve sessions individually, in group, or a mixture) and is highly problem focused. Sessions are structured to examine and change the negative beliefs. Homework is given for the problem thoughts and reactions.

CBT can be a critical method for relapse prevention. Its utility and effectiveness call for its greater dissemination and use.

Group Therapy, Including Relapse Prevention and Social Skills Training

Complementary to CBT is group therapy, offered in a variety of professional and lay settings. Group approaches to substance use disorders may be more effective than individual therapy because of the power of peers and their capacity to better respond to minimization, denial, and negative thinking.

Relapse prevention groups are particularly essential. Substance use disorders are chronic, relapsing conditions. We have to expect relapse. Patients, families, and clinicians can work to reduce its incidence. This approach began in the 1970s, led by Dr. Alan Marlatt. The approach stresses learning skills that can counteract a person's specific vulnerabilities to relapse, including craving, loneliness, emotional stress, peer pressure, and physical drivers such as fatigue and hunger.

The US Substance Abuse and Mental Health Services Administration (SAMHSA) includes relapse prevention in its registry of evidence-based programs for substance use disorders.

Skill-building groups that teach and practice interpersonal and communication skills provide participants with alternatives to "saying yes" to substances. They are similar in their approach to relapse prevention, and their provision is vital.

Look for programs or services that deliver skill training and relapse prevention; ask about it—insist upon it. These are different from 12-step programs and complement a host of other recovery efforts.

Contingency Management

Contingency management has had its detractors. It means pairing a desired behavior, such as abstinence, with a reward. Some have said, "Why pay people to be abstinent?" and "Besides, where would the money come from anyway?" But over time, evidence has been quite strong that rewarding people for staying clean and sober works. This includes not only financial rewards, but also tokens or movie tickets, vouchers, or prize drawings; even AA gives its members symbolic, inexpensive tokens for achieving milestones of sobriety. With contingency management, people with substance use problems are rewarded for clean urine, and their attendance at clinical visits improves.

Negative contingencies can work as well, such as loss of privileges in a group home for people with addictions or shunning or blaming by family members. But, again and again, we know from too many psychological studies that rewards are far more enduring than punishments. And they are more humane as well.

One thing about contingency management must be understood: if the incentives are discontinued, the effect diminishes over time. But then again, the effects of most treatments that are stopped for chronic conditions reduce over time.

Family Education and Skill Building

In the chapter on prevention, I discussed how targeted efforts with families, especially for youth, can prevent both the onset of problem drinking and drug use as well as serve as a component of early intervention. (This is also known as *secondary prevention*—a term for efforts made early on after a problem has emerged.)

For youth, even later in their adolescence, but certainly for those below the age of fourteen or fifteen, most (but not all) families remain great influencers of their children's behaviors. The younger the child is, the more influence the family usually has, since peers soon gain hegemony in the lives of teenagers. Parents can model responsible behaviors, including the moderate use of alcohol, build their bonds with their children through acquired and practiced communication techniques, and learn ways to set and reinforce family rules. Having family dinners regularly, and not in front of the TV, is a basic and invaluable way for families to effectively live with and respect one another. Even former president Barack Obama, for his eight years in the White House, had dinner with his wife and two daughters each evening (when possible!) at six thirty.

For people with developed substance use disorders, including adults, families remain the greatest and most enduring source of emotional, practical, and financial support. Excluding families is bad for patients, families, and for clinicians who want to succeed.

The phone message from my patient Eleanor Long, a mother in her forties now living in a Southern state, asked if I could speak right away. I called her later that day.

She was urgently concerned about her nineteen-year-old daughter, who had begun college in a New England city. An older brother, also living in the same city, had called to say that his sister, Andrea, was no longer going to classes. What's worse, she had a live-in boyfriend, a drug dealer, and they were using drugs and alcohol in what her brother described as a seemingly endless binge.

The family was affluent; they had set up Andrea with a comfortable apartment near the campus, gave her generous limits on her credit cards, and paid her tuition and all the usual college expenses. But she was using their money to cover her deepening descent into addiction.

Andrea did not suffer neglect or abuse as a child, nor did she live in a dangerous neighborhood. Her biological father likely had a mood disorder, perhaps bipolar illness, used marijuana heavily, and was emotionally volatile and threatening. Her mother was competent and devoted to her children, giving them opportunities to pursue their talents and dreams. The family was financially secure. While Andrea had the risk factor of mental illness and substance use in her biological family, her protective factors were substantial, likely keeping her from using drugs until she was away at school. These factors most likely helped tip the balance toward her recovery, but not right away.

Eleanor and I spoke over the ensuing days about her daughter, addictive behaviors, and where this might lead. We came to understand that Eleanor, as a mom, had two choices. One was to express great concern and try to reason with her daughter to get help and protect herself from the dangers of her behavior, while continuing her generous allowance. The other was to make ongoing financial support contingent on Andrea's getting treatment, working toward a clean and sober life, keeping a limited school schedule, and parting ways with those involved in drugs, including her drug-using boyfriend.

Whether to stand by and unconditionally support or to use what leverage (conditional support) they had was the toughest decision this family ever had to make, knowing they were between the proverbial rock and a hard (drug) place. It was not an easy choice for me, either, as their doctor.

What if they continued to support her, no matter what, and a medical or legal disaster ensued from her behavior? What if they decided to make their support contingent and she disappeared from their lives until they got a nightmarish call from a morgue—one that would haunt me as well? In the end, this case of family and individual treatment was a success. Not all are, and some take considerably more time before safety and normalcy return.

Eleanor and her second husband briefly tried the first option, offering Andrea support with no consequences for her continued drug use. But they knew soon from their son, the landlord, and the school that it wasn't working. They got lots of promises from Andrea, in the few calls that she answered, but she continued to live one dazed day to the next.

They feared the second choice, for good reason. A person in the throes of addiction, facing withdrawal and the work of rebuilding a life, will do most anything to keep the intoxication going and withdrawal at bay. I knew that and believed that reasoning with someone deep into his or her addiction has its (considerable) limits. Eleanor feared that if the family cut off Andrea's credit, which was funding the addiction—as was the drug dealing by her boyfriend—she could likely turn to getting money the old-fashioned way, by prostitution. If they ended rent payments, she could become homeless. They also imagined her wrath and potential alienation from their lives.

For nearly two months, the family, with my involvement, struggled to decide. In their hearts and minds, they knew that they would get nowhere with pleading and hanging their hopes on false promises. I thought they should opt for contingency: offer to pay for all that was in Andrea's interest (such as school, treatment, a home free of criminality), but halt her credit and then rent if she did not get with the program. But that carried the grave risk of its not working, as well as their having to brace themselves for their daughter's possible explosive reaction. I was open with my opinion but explicit that they had to decide and be able to live with the outcome should it be catastrophic. Her parents soon realized that time was not on their side. Addiction carries with it daily threats, and longer-term risks of physical disease, toxicity to the brain and harm to cognitive capabilities, and messy legal problems. I supported the decision to set clear and supportive limits and deeply hoped it would work.

Steeling herself, Eleanor visited Andrea to confront her in person. After some difficulty finding her, Eleanor expressed a love that could not stand by and watch this self-destruction. Eleanor laid out the rules for support and a plan for treatment that we had set up in advance.

Andrea's first response was not a surprise; we had rehearsed for that moment. I had asked Eleanor to practice with me what she would say when her daughter accused her of not loving her, as I imagined she would. How could Eleanor not get undone, give in, or get angry? She needed to say many, many times that she loved her daughter, and that love was at the core of what Eleanor was doing. I had asked Eleanor what she would say when her daughter said she hated Eleanor. Nothing may have been the best answer, but it is truly hard to be silent at a moment such as that. I had asked how Eleanor would respond to the pleading, to more of the same promises. It might be hard for her to not be curt and say she was tired of the same story—or that she had been disappointed too many times. What she needed to say was she believed in Andrea and thought the way to rebuild was the one Eleanor was asking her to take. I asked what Eleanor would say, and feel, if her daughter threatened to never see her again or, more frighteningly, threatened suicide or something otherwise dangerous. Each of these likely and heartrending emotional assaults called for not giving in, and not trying to bargain. This was going to be hard. Eleanor's conviction and faith in doing what was right had to steady her.

When they met, I learned that a stream of pleading, blaming, hating, and threatening was followed by Andrea's dramatic exit from the room. She could not be found for one day, then a second. Eleanor, with considerable support, stayed the course. Inside, she was churning, fearing the worst, and trying to bear the fiery accusation that she could not love her daughter and treat her this way.

After two months Andrea went for her first appointment with a therapist who would work with her on her co-occurring addiction and depression. That happened just before the clock was about to run out on the rent. What happened to the boyfriend was not clear to me, but he appeared to be gone. It was a good year before Andrea achieved some significant sobriety, was attending classes, and spoke regularly with her family. Almost another year passed before she offered her first thanks to them. Now, years later, this chapter in their family's life is painfully memorable, but it is past.

Andrea was using substances because her body craved them, because of being taken over by the disease, mind and body. Andrea's mother, with the support of her second husband and other children, and with my coaching, had decided it was a necessary gamble to cut Andrea off. This family's decision proved successful, but it was a gamble nonetheless. A therapist such as me has to have informed opinions and be willing to voice them, but let the patient and family decide what to do.

A family is usually the greatest support and ally that a person with a mental illness, including an addiction, can have. The decisions a family has to make about their loved one's mental health are not easy, nor are they cut-and-dried, and the results are not predictable. Families can both see the early-warning signs of trouble and be an essential source of love and hope through the demands and doubts that derive from these conditions. Many times, families help pay for costly and long-term treatments, sometimes mortgaging what little they have. I am reminded by my work with Eleanor that it is family, and friends, who gives rise to the saying that those who go the furthest in recovering from illness do not do so alone.

Community Reinforcement and Family Training (CRAFT) is a valuable resource for families developed by Dr. Robert Meyers. His work begins with recognizing the value of most families (and friends) in enabling a person with a substance use disorder to begin the work of recovery.

CRAFT is described by the American Psychological Association as a tool for families with a member who abuses alcohol or drugs. The CRAFT approach has been effective with different types of substance users, as well as across family relationship types (e.g., parent-child, sibling, etc.) and among different ethnicities.

This approach benefits both the person with an addiction, helping him or her to engage in treatment even after family members have had as few as five sessions of CRAFT, *and* the families themselves, who report feeling less depressed and less angry. The families also experience reduced conflict and greater cohesion—even if the affected family member has yet to enter treatment. This approach assumes that while most families mean well, they may lack the tools to do well. Families are urged to understand their emotional states;

their motivation to help their loved one; their optimism or pessimism; and their level of self-care, since they need to take care of themselves if they are to effectively care for a loved one. Clear goals for self-care—for instance, getting sleep, proper nutrition, and time with other loved ones—for family members and even clearer responses to reinforce healthy behaviors in a loved one are developed, practiced, and monitored to help ensure their adoption both early on and in the ongoing work of sustaining recovery.

The CRAFT approach stresses collaboration, not conflict; it stresses kindness, not confrontation. It enlists a person's motivation to change by seeking to understand how the addictive behavior is rewarding to the user, how the drug use serves a purpose—even if it is not doing so effectively. From there, the approach helps the user build alternative activities and strategies to tap into similar, but healthier, rewards.

Medication-Assisted Treatment (MAT)

The use of medications that diminish cravings, reduce relapses, and enable people to escape a life of compulsively pursuing drugs can be controversial in the recovery community. Some 12-step philosophies are explicitly against the use of psychoactive substances even for these purposes, especially opioids and tranquilizers. I recall decades ago when these programs were against the use of antipsychotic, mood-stabilizing, and antidepressant medications. While that opposition to medications for co-occurring psychiatric conditions has largely abated—and 12-step programs never proclaimed the "dangers" of insulin or antihypertensives—the use of MAT causes much ambivalence, especially among counselors who gained their recovery with an abstinence-only approach.

I don't consider the host of medications used to treat co-occurring mental and physical diseases to be treatments for substance use disorders. Instead, medications such as antidepressants, mood stabilizers, and antipsychotic agents are specific therapies for the other conditions that quite frequently occur in people with a substance use disorder, not unlike insulin for diabetes. MAT specifically targets, instead, an element of the addictive response in the brain.

I believe substance-dependent individuals should seek a program that includes the opportunity for MAT. While medications are not for everyone, reduced rates of relapse and improved function (not to mention eschewing a life of crime) are among the key benefits of MAT.

Three types of medication can be used for opioid dependence. They are not always mutually exclusive and include agonists (medications that enhance the activity of opioids at specific neurotransmitter sites, additive to our natural neurotransmitters) such as methadone and buprenorphine; antagonists such as naloxone and Vivitrol, which counter the actions of opioids in the brain; and other agents. Agonists activate an existing brain neuronal receptor, effecting a response, while antagonists are their opposite, blocking the action of the substance at the nerve receptor sites.

Agonists

Methadone is an opioid agonist, acting principally on and fully occupying the μ-opioid receptor in the brain. Though methadone was developed in Germany in the late 1930s, it did not find general use in the United States until the early 1960s, as a result of the groundbreaking work done at Rockefeller University by Drs. Vincent Dole and Marie Nyswander. The uses of methadone include analgesia (pain relief), detoxification from other opioids, and maintenance, in which a person takes daily doses, as part of a treatment program. It is usually taken by mouth as a pill, sublingually, or in a liquid, but can also be injected for acute pain relief; effects last up to one full day when used for regular maintenance.

Methadone produces both tolerance and dependence, the latter more so for long-term maintenance users. Because it is a full agonist, high doses can flood brain receptors, rendering a user unconscious and depressing breathing, thereby potentially causing respiratory arrest and death. For some people, methadone maintenance is lifesaving. It can rescue families and communities from emotional hardship as well as high health-care and correctional-system costs; but for some individuals, particularly if it is mixed with alcohol, tranquilizers, or other opioids, it can cause overdose and death.

For people with a persistent dependence on opioids, particularly high doses of heroin and prescription pain pills, and who need a highly structured program, methadone remains a mainstay MAT.

Buprenorphine became legal in the United States in 2000 and available a few years later, after a long, puritanical federal inquisition about its introduction. When it was released for medical prescribing, I was mental health (including the addictions) commissioner in New York City and saw the availability of this drug as vital to providing scores of thousands of New Yorkers an alternative to street drugs *and* to methadone maintenance programs, which many addicts did not want to use. Over a decade later its use remains limited, especially in light of its relative safety and the extent of the opioid epidemic.

Buprenorphine simultaneously acts as a partial agonist to the opioid receptor and as an antagonist. It is far more difficult to get high or overdose on this agent, unless it is mixed with other, non-opioid substances that depress the central nervous system such as tranquilizers or alcohol. Buprenorphine binds fiercely to receptors, thus blocking the uptake of (or receptor displacement by) other opioids, making ingestion of heroin, methadone, or opioid analgesics usually not worth the effort. The two principal preparations are Subutex, which contains only buprenorphine, and Suboxone, which compounds the buprenorphine with naloxone to deter its injection. (Withdrawal would immediately ensue from the injected, but not orally taken, naloxone. Naloxone is an opioid full antagonist in the brain. If a person takes naloxene, any opioid activity in the brain [and body] will be fully blocked, inducing a state of immediate and distressing withdrawal.)

Patients can be prescribed buprenorphine for up to a thirty-day supply (and there is now a long-acting preparation, described below) by physicians who take a course and obtain certification to use this medication. Patients do not need to go daily to a methadone clinic and can have their privacy more protected by seeing a primary-care physician. Because of the convenience and the reportedly less sedating action of buprenorphine compared to methadone, many experience greater functioning, including competitive employment. At first, physicians could serve only 30 active cases; then the number, with additional approval, became 100. Regulatory changes have now increased that number to 275, over time (with perhaps 500 in the future), as well as now permitting trained nurse practitioners to prescribe in order to improve access to this medication.

Through most of the period of its medical use, diversion of buprenorphine was limited. However, more recently this drug has gained greater street value; it has become a type of "insurance" for opioid users in the event they cannot obtain their usual opioid supply or want to withdraw to reduce their tolerance (and thus the cost of their habit). Preparations have diversified as well; first came the sublingual pill, then the dissolvable film, and most recently a set of four tiny sustained-release implants under the skin that can last up to six months.

Buprenorphine can be a critical, lifesaving, and life-producing MAT for people with opioid addiction. Its safety, utility, and convenience make it an important option—yet one still highly underused.

Antagonists

Naloxone and Vivitrol are the most employed and useful opioid antagonists.

Naloxone is first and foremost a lifesaver. EMTs, police, and, increasingly, friends and families of people using opioids carry a vial or two of naloxone nasal spray to use if someone overdoses. Countless lives have already been saved. Naloxone preparations also include intramuscular and auto-injection syringes. It acts immediately and effectively, reversing respiratory arrest and loss of consciousness. It is like the automatic defibrillator of the addiction world.

Naltrexone, a variant of naloxone in pill form, has been used to reduce cravings as well as the rewarding effects of alcohol and drugs. Its relatively new and important utility is in its monthly intramuscular preparation, Vivitrol, which, though costly, can be worth the price for its ability to reduce harm and help toward achieving abstinence.

Other Agents

Acamprosate has had limited uptake among treatment providers and patients, suggesting its limited effectiveness. This drug is believed to modulate or inhibit brain glutamate receptors, thereby diminishing a drug-dependent person's need to mitigate (by using again) withdrawal discomfort, which induces craving and relapse.

NAC (N-acetylcysteine) is available from your local Walmart, CVS, or online. Sold as a nutraceutical, or dietary supplement, it also has effects on glutamate and dopamine transmission in the brain. It may reduce inflammation, a ubiquitous cause of cellular and organ dysfunction. NAC has been used with cannabis addiction and a number of psychiatric disorders. It is quite safe and not costly, but it is not covered by third-party insurance payers.

Disulfiram is the old man of addiction treatment. I recall prescribing it, rather unsuccessfully, decades ago. It still exists and is sometimes prescribed, though it is not much sought after. If people take this medication and then drink alcohol, they will soon become sick—nauseated, vomiting, sweating, and tremulous. It is meant to be a deterrent, but if people want to drink, they merely need to stop taking it and wait a couple of days. With a supportive and attentive family it can be more effective. Because disulfiram increases brain dopamine, some have considered it a potential treatment (an agonist) for stimulant addiction.

Meditation, Exercise, and Diet

Alternatives to and treatments for substance abuse overlap a lot, especially in the realms of meditation, mindfulness, and yoga; exercise; and diet. A variety of mind-body practices can deliver immense benefits for people with substance use disorder, and just about every other chronic disorder. With addiction, for instance, mindfulness may help a person experiencing a craving observe that craving, appreciate its transitory nature, and accept the feeling, thereby resisting acting on it. I have personally used mindfulness, including breathing and stress-reduction techniques, in the wake of disasters in my public mental health work—specifically, those techniques taught by Drs. Richard Brown and Patricia Gerbarg, two of the foremost medical practitioners and teachers of complementary and alternative medicine. Their best-known book, with Dr. Philip Muskin, *How to Use Herbs, Nutrients, and*

Yoga in Mental Health Care, is clear, concise, comprehensive, and helpful. Their even more recent book, *Complementary and Integrative Treatments in Psychiatric Practice*, gives us a fine look at a host of alternative treatments that educates readers about existing and emerging therapeutic options and how they work.

Exercise, another way to forge a healthy mind-body connection, can make perhaps the greatest difference in our health, well-being, longevity, memory, and stamina. If anyone could compound exercise into a pill, it would vastly outsell Cialis, Viagra, and Lipitor together.

I can imagine referring a person with a substance use problem or depression to Vincenz Priessnitz—though he, alas, died in 1851. Priessnitz was a pioneer in alternative medicine, gaining fame throughout Europe, America, and as far as New Zealand for curing his patients by combining baths with vigorous exercise, adequate sleep, and proper diet. His recommended form of exercise, called the walking cure, consisted of long walks in fresh air, barefoot when the season permitted. It fits well with modern medicine, which indicates that a sedentary lifestyle invites chronic inflammation throughout the body, a key factor in depression, addictions, autoimmune disorders, and cardiovascular and neurodegenerative illnesses. Exercise ups our body's metabolic rate and improves our sense of well-being; can release endorphins, the closest thing to opioids we naturally produce; and can reduce stress levels and stress hormones. Through exercise, dopamine binding is increased, glutamate is decreased, and brain plasticity is enhanced.

Diet is another important factor in well-being, especially for people with addictions. For those with long-standing substance dependence, their diet must be carefully shaped to provide nutrients, vitamins, and minerals that may have been depleted by their use of drugs, poverty, and a horrific lifestyle. People less depleted by substance use still require a balanced diet—even, for some, a Mediterranean, Paleo, or vegan lifestyle—as an essential part of the foundation for health and recovery. As my good friend Dr. Drew Ramsey says, "The best prescription is at the end of a fork."

Psychedelic Agents and Recovery

Earlier we discussed the use of LSD, psilocybin, and other mind-altering agents as tools for treatment of pain, depression, and possibly even PTSD and addiction. Some limited evidence suggests that someday, with more of the right research, we may see psychedelic agents, or derivative drugs, used for mental illness and addiction treatment.

In 2017, Ayelet Waldman published a journal describing her use of microdoses of LSD, ten micrograms from a dropper instead of one hundred or more on a blotter, which was not enough to produce hallucinations but did profoundly impact her chronic, treatment-resistant depression. She called the book *A Really Good Day* to signify how she came to feel after decades of malaise. She presented the treatment plan she adopted, off the beaten path, but she had tried every other path.

Each day's report is far more than a journal of drug effects. The reader is treated to a thoughtful, sometimes even humorous, perspective on the history of drugs in this country, the neuroscience of psychedelics and stimulants, the injustices perpetrated against people of color because of the criminalization of psychoactive drugs, how to talk with your kids about life (including drugs), the powerful public-health concept of harm reduction, and so much more by this public defender, law professor, student of history, and wise and suffering person.

The LSD worked for her—and though we know that a case report of one does not science make, material dates back to the

1960s on the potential for psychedelic drugs to not only open us up to wonder but to pull us out of despair and possibly addiction. Despite our country's unhelpful puritanical ethos, research is picking up. Someday, we may be prescribing microdoses of LSD or a couple psilocybin trips (or similar agents) for people with addictions, pain, and other chronic, debilitating conditions.

Harm Reduction

For many years, public-health doctors and government officials have recognized that the morbidity a disease produces (suffering, physical and emotional distress, and the use of expensive medical care) can be mitigated by interventions. These are known as harm-reduction strategies.

For example, when people with drug addictions use syringes, these can produce even greater problems than the drug itself. HIV and hepatitis C are readily spread by shared or dirty syringes. The harm-reduction strategy is to provide clean syringes, at accessible neighborhood sites, in "exchange" for used syringes. These sites also seek to connect people in need with treatment. As another example, sexually transmitted diseases such as syphilis, gonorrhea, herpes, and AIDS are readily spread by unprotected sex. The harm-reduction strategy is to supply condoms, free and just about everywhere (in bathrooms, schools, and clinics). Both of these strategies are highly effective and have generally overcome arguments to simply not use drugs or to forgo sex.

I recently consulted on a young man in his early twenties, let's call him John, who had been in a psychiatric hospital unit for many weeks. This was his fourth admission in the past year and a half. Able doctors, nurses, psychologists, and social workers had been trying hard to quiet his paranoid ideas and frightened and at times aggressive mental states. From childhood he had been diagnosed as having autistic spectrum disorder (ASD), on the higher end of functioning—what had not long ago been termed Asperger's syndrome. He had not only odd, idiosyncratic thinking but also great difficulty being around other people. He preferred to be alone, could not make eye contact, and generally needed a familiar, highly repetitive daily schedule. He often lost himself in video games for hours on end, which seemed the greatest of his pleasures, along with smoking marijuana, daily when he could afford it. He lived in a state where recreational cannabis was legal.

John also developed a co-occurring psychotic illness in late adolescence. It resembled schizophrenia, a persistent, serious mental illness with impairments in social and cognitive functioning as well as delusions and hallucinations. I say resembled because people with ASD can develop psychotic states whose symptoms can appear the same as those of schizophrenia, but which generally call for a somewhat different therapeutic approach. The psychotic symptoms, with delusions of being controlled, of having great powers, and of fearing for his safety, destabilized John and resulted in his being brought to emergency services and admitted to a hospital unit.

His treatment team had tried recognized approaches to his psychotic symptoms, starting with antipsychotic medications and efforts to engage him in counseling. His family was engaged but was at a distance. But his condition did not improve. He frequently refused medication and became agitated when asked to speak with staff or to join treatment groups. One unsuccessful medication trial led to another, and to the addition of a second class of drugs called mood stabilizers with the thought they might help quiet his labile moods. Nothing was working, and he was retreating more into himself, thus the request for consultation.

My thoughts were counterintuitive to the conventional medical approaches the inpatient professional staff had been using, in part because these approaches were not working. I also believe that while inpatient care can at times be necessary, it also can foster loss of everyday functioning and, for some people, trigger further loss of reality testing as they lose control of their everyday activities to the hospital's institutional demands. I suggested that perhaps the staff had done what they could and that they should say to John they wanted to work with him toward a prompt discharge. I added that he would never take psychiatric medications after he left the hospital because he did not think he needed them, nor did he think they had any benefit, only side effects. I believed he would return to the two measures that gave him the greatest psychic relief, cannabis and video games, and that not only should the staff expect him to resume these immediately, but they should not oppose his doing so.

The reactions in the conference room to my suggestions were pretty mixed. People were also appropriately concerned about his leaving while still in an actively psychotic state; he could be at risk for exposure to the elements, staying out all night poorly dressed, or getting frightened on the street and striking a stranger. All true, I said. But we had no reason to believe that doing more of the same would have a different outcome. What's more, I believed that the intense milieu of the hospital with all its social demands could be making John worse. He had the neurobiology of a person with ASD and needed to be in control of his environment and to limit his exposure to other people. And he was without the two self-selected activities that brought him the most comfort, cannabis and video games.

I added that I would urge him to buy cannabis with 40 percent cannabidiol, or near to it, which would be available to him. As noted earlier, cannabidiol is a common ingredient in cannabis, though THC is the most common and what produces the high. Cannabidiol does not produce a high and seems to be protective against the psychotic symptoms that THC can produce, especially in vulnerable and adolescent brains. Research is under way to see if cannabidiol can be medicinally used as an antipsychotic.

My consultation with John employed two harm-reduction strategies. First, I recognized that John had ready access to marijuana and would use it. No one was going to talk him out of that—nor of his resuming gaming when he was out from under the control of a hospital setting. Patient preferences are well-known to good clinicians because we all are far more apt to do what we want than what others want from us. I was urging the clinical staff to hew to his intention to use by adopting a harm-reduction strategy by recommending a form of cannabis that might be less toxic to his brain.

The second harm-reduction strategy was a bit more atypical. I was working from the premise that the hospital setting was worsening his mental state, activating more anxiety and loss of control. The more time in the hospital, the more medical staff running his life, the more at risk he was for further regression. I told the group the story of Philippe Pinel, who legendarily took the mental patients out of their chains in a Paris asylum in the late 1700s; they did better when freed. Not that John was literally in chains, but that might well be his psychic experience.

All medical interventions must weigh and balance risk and benefit. That was the calculus the staff I consulted with needed to employ. There was risk in his staying in the hospital, and there was risk in his leaving. There was risk in his resuming smoking cannabis, and there was risk in his refraining since he knew this was the most effective anxiolytic for him (as was video gaming). I hoped this talented and dedicated hospital staff would see that the benefits of harm reduction could outweigh the risks. Taking care of patients is a privilege, and it can be hard because often the stakes are high.

Transcranial Magnetic Stimulation (TMS)

We are just getting started with magnetic-stimulation treatments for a variety of mental and addictive disorders. The low toxicity and safety of TMS calls for far more research and use of these new technologies.

TMS does not pass electricity into the brain, as does ECT. Instead, this noninvasive procedure passes an electromagnetic field through the skull into a person's brain. Scientists think its effects are on brain circuits, with their respective effects on neurotransmitters such as dopamine and glutamate. For most people, TMS is far better tolerated than medications. Repetitive TMS, or rTMS, is already an approved method for people whose depression does not respond to conventional treatments. Reports of the use of TMS for tobacco, stimulant, and alcohol addiction are also promising.

Policy Interventions: Prescription Drug Monitoring Programs (PDMPs) and Drug Courts

Prescription drug monitoring programs have been adopted by most states in an effort to control the medical prescription of opioids by doctors. PDMPs are developed and required by government regulators: pharmacies must report to a designated state agency on all doctors prescribing opioids, tranquilizers, and sedatives, and at what doses—letting doctors know that the state is watching. Thirty-nine states, including my own state of New York, have adopted PDMPs.

The data collected can help states to fashion targeted education programs as well as to identify and intervene with doctors whose prescribing patterns suggest that they are "pill mills," conveying to too many patients, collectively, massive doses of controlled drugs, making a lot of money for the provider. The databases also allow doctors to know if one of their patients is receiving the same medication from another doctor, or many, as people dependent on opioids often go "doctor shopping."

Many states now require specific prescription forms or only permit electronic ordering of medications. These mandates complement the PDMPs. In some jurisdictions, the number of pills that can be prescribed, especially for initial prescriptions for acute pain, is limited (e.g., a seven-day supply), and a new prescription, not a refill, is required for further medication, unlike for many other drugs such as heart medications, antidepressants, and blood-sugar control agents.

Across the country, we have seen in recent years significant reductions in the prescription of opioid medications. In my public appearances, on radio and in community talks, many patients with chronic pain that had been on these drugs have voiced concerns that their doctors won't give them the medication they need and have used, nonabusively, for years. Such is one unintended and unfortunate consequence of surveillance of doctors: *inappropriate* prescribing may be reduced as well as *appropriate* prescribing. The pendulum may have swung a bit too far from where it was and may take time to swing back to what might be regarded as equipoise.

Critics of PDMPs (as a singular solution) also note that while opioid prescriptions are down, overdose deaths continue to rise.

However, that appears to be related to the growth in illegal use of opioids, including of pills fabricated abroad, and users' progression to heroin and fentanyl—and fentanyl's more novel forms, which are far more deadly drugs than the others.

Drug courts are another useful policy intervention. Eligible drug-addicted persons may be sent to drug court, in lieu of the traditional justice system, and be directed to long-term treatment under close supervision. For a minimum term of one year, participants are provided with intensive treatment and other services to help them get and stay clean and sober; are held accountable by the drug court judge for meeting their obligations to the court, society, themselves, and their families; are regularly and randomly tested for drug use; are required to appear in court frequently so that a judge may review their progress; and are supported for doing well or sanctioned when they do not meet their obligations.

Drug courts work. Seventy-five percent of those who complete the adult court program are never arrested again. The first drug court was started in 1989 in Miami-Dade County, Florida, and there are now close to three thousand drug courts nationally—but far fewer than needed to serve the estimated 1.2 million drug-addicted individuals caught up in our criminal justice system, just another instance of the persistence of correctional-system approaches to addiction despite more effective and humane alternatives.

Stay the Course
With addictions, and chronic diseases of all sorts, staying with treatment and building a healthier lifestyle is hard work. With substances, relapse is to be expected, prevented when possible, and always responded to with support, vigor, and hope.

While we know that great numbers of people with substance use disorders recover, we are not good at predicting when. That calls for staying the course, dusting ourselves off, and having a go at it again as soon as possible when relapse darkens the door. Everyone needs to believe that recovery is possible. Everyone needs to work to keep hope alive.

Addiction spares no one because of age, gender, race, privilege, or social status. In a pair of interviews in *Glamour* magazine and the *Today* show, Christina Huffington, the daughter of prominent spokesperson and now former *Huffington Post* editor in chief Arianna Huffington, told the all-too-familiar story of the progression of the disease of addiction until she was living on the knife's edge of life.

For Christina Huffington, her road to addiction began at age twelve, with surreptitious use of alcohol. By the time she began boarding at an East Coast prep school, she was drinking compulsively and showing signs of, in her words, "binge eating"—another compulsive behavior that led to admission to an eating-disorder program and a return to living closer to home. Then, at age sixteen, came that moment that people with addiction so frequently describe: the experience of using a substance and then feeling as they never had before, a feeling that seemed to demand repeating, and repeating and repeating.

Cocaine became her drug of choice, an expression in the addiction community that describes the one drug that a drug-dependent person prefers more than any other. She denied having a problem (another feature of the disease, especially early on and with no treatment) and stopped after she was caught at home. But she did not stop being an addict; she just stopped using for the moment. She worked hard at school, getting into Yale, and was clean for three years until she took the next snort. It was as if not a moment had passed; she was again as compulsive, and secretive, a user as she had been. Going from zero to sixty right away is also characteristic of addiction. Everything else gives way to using. She developed tolerance and a host of physical problems from her daily drug abuse. Finally, she got scared and told her mother. That is the first step in recovery: admitting you have a problem.

The next step was rehab, the beginning of a journey of recovery, which demands exploration of why the person was using the drug in the first place. Rehab is also the beginning of turning to others for support, and not only to stay sober—though that is essential. Many people in recovery, though not all, follow the 12-step approach familiar to many from AA, NA, and Al-Anon. Rehab can help patients learn to live a drug-free life, one in which love, work, and purpose serve as the natural highs we all need. For sure, the first time in rehab is not the one that works for many people. It can take a number of tries at being clean and sober, at living a life of recovery, before the process fully takes hold. Experienced clinicians know not to give up hope even though it can be hard to predict when recovery will really kick in; people with addiction, and their families, need to know this as well to stay the course, to persist and be there when a person wants to try again.

What we don't want to see or admit, we do not remedy. Within a family and within our culture, tackling addiction starts with detecting it. Simple screening tests for alcohol, drugs, and tobacco exist and can be made standard practice throughout medical care (and in educational and counseling settings). SBIRT—Screening, Brief Intervention, and Referral to Treatment, discussed earlier in this book—is a recognized, proven, and even reimbursed medical procedure that awaits general use despite the consequences we suffer from not using it.

People may take many different paths to addiction recovery. No one path works for everyone. Community Reinforcement and Family Training (CRAFT), noted earlier, is a valuable resource for families developed by Dr. Robert Meyers. His work begins with recognizing the value of most families (and friends) in enabling a person with a substance use disorder to begin the work of recovery.

For some, 12-step programs are lifesaving. Others benefit from medications that aid in remaining drug-free (as noted earlier, medication-assisted treatment, or MAT) coupled with psychotherapy. We all, not just addicts, need to surround ourselves with people who want to support our well-being, and to assiduously avoid people who want to exploit and otherwise take advantage of us.

Addiction remains America's most neglected disease. When celebrities, sports figures, and political leaders go public about their addictions, that helps diminish stigma and foster hope, just as the Huffingtons did.

There are an abundance of treatments for addiction, and no shoe fits all feet; many interventions are usually better than just one or two. With complex problems, which surely include substance use disorders, we have to use a lot of good stuff, heartily applied over time, to increase the chances of success. The road begins by walking it.

7

WHAT COMES NEXT

Research is creating new knowledge.
—NEIL ARMSTRONG

Research is what I'm doing when I don't know what I'm doing.
—WERNHER VON BRAUN

The field of addictions faces an extraordinary nexus of challenges. Substance abuse and dependence involves genetics; environment; experience; social values; neural molecules, transmitters, and circuits; cognition; personality; and other vectors. While science has increasingly good clues about the progression from substance use to compulsive use and addiction, Wernher von Braun reminds us that there is always more we don't understand.

In my work as a public-health doctor, I seek to understand and promote three types of research: basic science, translational research, and services research, akin to program evaluation.

In basic-science efforts, studied guesses (hypotheses) are subjected to the rigorous proofs of science. Work in basic science includes biological and cognitive neuroscience studies into how our brains and minds work; how they are changed by internal and external events; and how to take action to promote desired changes. Neurological molecular elements and physiological processes are all part of basic neuroscience. From time to time, often through serendipity or because an alert scientist notes something unexpected, there is discovery, new knowledge.

New knowledge, however, can take a long time to be applied. How might evidence of, say, down regulation (dampening) of dopamine receptors inform our understanding of the pathogenesis of addiction and direct our therapeutic efforts? How can cognitive neuroscience, with its clear demonstration of the power of cues (conditioned responses), be used to help people with addictions? Here, we use translational research to understand how knowledge can be "translated" into practice. The so-called science-to-practice gap is the often exceptionally long time before knowledge becomes standard practice—for instance, achieving systematic hand washing in hospitals or detection of substance and mental disorders in primary care. Translational research aims to highlight the best bridges from research to clinical care.

My state government work includes oversight of two sizable and successful psychiatric research institutes, yet I still believe that the greatest gains in the next five to ten years will come from doing more of what we know works and from translating what we know into what we actually do daily. While this involves translational research, in many cases it also calls for services research.

We know, for example, that buprenorphine can fill craving opioid brain receptors, but for which patients, at what point in their addictions, with which medical distribution channels, and with what associated programming can it work best? Who will be better served by methadone as a medication-assisted treatment? For whom and where will relapse prevention groups work best, and for how long? Will mindfulness help as an addition to a substance use program, and if so, how can it best be delivered? Can exercise reduce the need for medication of all types? What types of health insurance coverage can help people with substance problems, and what barriers exist to their provision? The more answers we have that can be demonstrated in vivo, in clinical and community settings during everyday patient care, the more likely we will see people with addictions and their families better served and resources most effectively employed. That is what services research can contribute.

Dr. Nora Volkow wrote in her inimitable way that addiction involves "the desensitization of reward circuits, which dampens the ability to feel pleasure and the motivation to pursue everyday activities; the increasing strength of conditioned responses and stress reactivity, which results in increased cravings . . . and negative emotions when these cravings are not sated; and the weakening of the brain regions involved in executive functions such as decision making, inhibitory control, and self-regulation that leads to repeated relapse." Each of the elements Dr. Volkow so concisely describes represents research opportunities to help those affected by these common and destructive diseases.

Addiction appears to follow a three-stage process. At first, use and abuse stimulate reward pathways and relieve physical and psychic pain. Users feel good and get relief from what ails them. But continued use can soon bring the dark side. As the acute effects of a persistently used drug wear off, the user feels withdrawn, fatigued, dulled to everyday life, depressed, and anxious, among other negative states—the second stage. When the disease progresses to the third stage, tolerance and dependence, users are continuously preoccupied with obtaining and using their substance of choice. Their lives revolve around the drug, with compulsive consumption, impulsive actions that dismiss bad consequences—such as family alienation, lost employment, financial ruin, and ill health—and relapse when they make efforts to stop. Each of these stages represents research opportunities to increase our knowledge and more effectively prevent, treat, and mitigate addiction.

In May 2016, I attended a two-day conference put on by the New York Academy of Sciences and the Aspen Brain Forum called the Addicted Brain and New Treatment Frontiers. I was impressed by the range and sophistication of neuroscience research under way, but nevertheless left thinking of all the work we still have to do. From that conference, my colleagues in addiction medicine and science, and reports I have studied, I will offer some areas where there are significant promising scientific investigations and more support is needed to achieve practical applications.

Eric Nestler, MD, at the Icahn School of Medicine and the Friedman Brain Institute in New York, has called addiction "drug-induced neural plasticity." This means that substance use changes brain cells and the way transmissions go from one cell to another, thereby changing the communication that goes on in the brain. Glutamate and GABA receptors, for example, are altered with addiction, producing measurable structural changes in the brain—that is, actual alterations in neural circuits. For example, learning and memory paths can be impaired; this is especially true of the adolescent brain, which we know to be "under construction" and thus highly vulnerable.

Vaccines may be one way to prevent this villainous plasticity in addiction. Vaccines are attenuated agents that prompt the body to create antibodies against those specific agents; think of influenza or polio vaccines. A vaccine might selectively create antibodies, for example, to cocaine, nicotine, heroin, or fentanyl that would bind to the specific drug used and block its action. This is like the world of immunotherapy, which holds promise for cancer and other diseases. Though no adequately effective vaccine has yet been produced, it may only be a matter of time.

Studies on primates have attached a virus (an adenovirus, such as the one for the common cold) to the drug of abuse selected—thereby using the virus as a Trojan horse to carry the drug of abuse, which will be fought by the body's natural defenses against the virus. The animal's liver can thus be stimulated to produce high titers of antibodies that are safe and lasting. A human vaccine study on people addicted to cocaine began in 2016. Vaccines could be used in high-risk individuals, those with family histories of addiction or living in dangerous environments. Vaccines could also be used with substance-dependent individuals with advanced diseases to help them stay clean and rebuild their lives.

Research on genetic variations may add precision to the selection of a medication-assisted treatment. As an example, in therapy for tobacco dependence, we have bupropion (Zyban) and varenicline (Chantix) to help smokers quit. But what if we could tell, say by genetic testing, which smokers are normal or fast or slow metabolizers of nicotine? That might make a difference in whether a person would do better with varenicline or bupropion or with a nicotine patch. Research is under way here as well.

We know that cortical controls are weakened by the chronic use of many substances, resulting in the diminution of executive functioning, including constraint and judgment. Might there be ways to stimulate specific areas, such as the prefrontal cortex, with light that activates certain genes (called optogenetic stimulation) to reduce the compulsive behaviors seen in addictions? Some promising work is under way in mice, which may point the way to its application in humans.

Transcranial magnetic stimulation (TMS), as discussed earlier, already has beneficial uses in people with severe depression. Might TMS energize the frontal lobes of people who have developed a reduced capacity to control impulses, thereby enabling them to think and thus behave in more adaptive ways? We do not yet know and need research to separate placebo effects from true therapeutic actions.

Deep brain stimulation (DBS), as well, has proven utility in Parkinson's disease and severe depression, as exemplified by the work of Dr. Helen Mayberg. Studies of rats administered DBS have shown transient improvements in their compulsive behaviors. Pairing DBS in these same animals with a dopamine antagonist not only helped behaviors, but was also associated with reversing cocaine-induced synaptic plasticity, which we have recognized as one of the basic pathogenic processes in addiction. This is science at its most miraculous, though it is basic research and still far from translation.

There has also been research into alleviating the effects of chronic stress, a terrible enemy to us humans. Chronic stress fosters compromised immunity, which leaves us at greater risk for infection and cancer. It also produces persistent levels of organ and blood-vessel inflammation, which promotes heart disease as well as stroke, diabetes, depression, arthritis, autoimmune diseases, PTSD, and many other chronic conditions. Chronic stress further does some of its deleterious work through the well-known hypothalamic–pituitary–adrenal axis (HPA).

The HPA axis is our internal governor, responding to and seeking to control stress reactions in the body. It is perhaps best known for the fight-or-flight reaction. But it also has a considerable role on our immune competence, through the release of cortisol and other corticosteroids; on our digestive processes; on libido; and on mood. The diagram on the next page shows the key elements of the HPA, and how their continuous feedback is meant to sustain homeostasis, or balance, in the body.

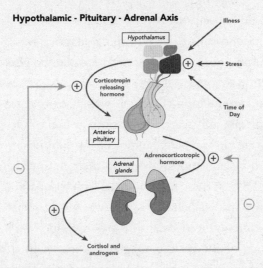

Hypothalamic - Pituitary - Adrenal Axis

The hypothalamic–pituitary–adrenal axis is our "internal governor" and controls the fight-or-flight response.

Chronic stress, and the chronic inflammation it produces, also release the corticotropin-releasing factor (CRF), which gears up the stress response, and dynorphin, an opioid peptide (protein) in our bodies that shuts down the dopamine system and leaves us feeling awful, and thus prone to seeking relief from drugs.

Drug abuse and dependence produce an increased reactivity to stress, which puts the user at high risk to relapse in order to abate feelings of heightened and persistent dysphoria. In the third stage of addiction, stress reactivity is high; drugs are principally employed for relief, not pleasure. (That is, unless you like Freud's definition of pleasure, which was the relief of pain.) Research into the brain's reward and stress systems—on how drug abuse attenuates the release of dopamine and makes life absent of feeling or deeply unpleasant from stress—is basic science meant to gain knowledge and direction for the field of substance and behavioral addictions.

However, because of the brain's immense complexity, cognitive neuroscience research may prove more immediately useful. CBT (cognitive behavioral therapy) and mindfulness techniques are showing considerable success in the lab and in translational and services research. Both these techniques can strengthen cortical executive functions and quiet the sympathetic (fight-or-flight) nervous system. CBT has already proven useful in relapse prevention because it can blunt a person's reverberations to cues, to reduce conditioned responses such as those produced by contact with friends who are using, social events where alcohol and drugs are readily accessible, and the insistent media fascination with drugs.

Program research has been active for many years on the use of medication-assisted treatment. Work has been especially prominent for nicotine and alcohol addictions, two of the principal causes of preventable morbidity and mortality in the United States and many other countries. Research into the use of opioid replacement medications (such as methadone and, more recently, buprenorphine, known as opioid agonists and discussed earlier) has shown that long-term gains can be achieved in opioid-dependent individuals. The work of my former colleague Dr. Roger Weiss, at McLean Hospital and Harvard Medical School, exemplifies these efforts. A three-and-a-half-year follow-up study of opioid-dependent individuals, the longest to date, demonstrated "marked improvements" in their use of illicit opioids and other substances when they were treated with opioid replacement agents. About 50 percent of study participants abstained from illicit opioid use in the months prior to the eighteen-month follow-up, and the rate increased to 60 percent by the end of the study. Participants also reported general improvements in their health and subjective pain.

Because of the prevalence of addiction in correctional settings, and substance-dependent individuals' great difficulty remaining clean and sober after release, services research into this population is essential. Relapse rates were lower in those treated with long-acting naltrexone (Vivitrol), but the positive effects abated when the medication was discontinued. The use of long-acting naltrexone, with its utility to reduce cravings, is another promising area of research for this group of high-risk individuals.

Research on the addictions, as we see from this group of examples, ranges from basic to translational to services research. Studies query genetics, molecules, circuits, cognition, prevention, and treatment—and who knows what lies ahead.

Complicated? Indeed.

A bit of science and science fiction? Maybe.

Promising? Hopefully.

Needed? Deeply.

8

THE PAINTED BIRD

No one is born hating another person because of the color of his skin, or his background, or his religion. People must learn to hate, and if they can learn to hate, they can be taught to love, for love comes more naturally to the human heart than its opposite.

—NELSON MANDELA

A boy wanders about Eastern Europe during World War II, fleeing the Nazis, who have captured his parents in Poland. So goes the remarkable tale in Jerzy Kosinski's book *The Painted Bird.* As the boy wanders, he witnesses an event where Kosinski's fiction gives us a clear window on truth. The boy comes upon a professional bird catcher who has painted a captured bird with many colors, then releases it to the sky. The boy watches as the soaring painted bird rejoins its flock—and is mercilessly attacked by its own. The bird plummets, dead, to the earth below.

At this moment when substance use, abuse, and dependence have achieved epidemic proportions in this and many other countries, it is time to revisit, understand, and revise the damaging views so commonly held about people with addictions. As great as the stigma of mental illness is, the ill will toward people with substance use disorders is even greater. The results of this stigma, and its co-traveler discrimination, are seen in the alienation and injustices these individuals experience; in the human pain and emotional burdens they and their families endure; in the excessive use of the correctional system, which disproportionately and unfairly impacts people living in poverty and of color; and in the wasteful expenditures of money and resources to fight a "war" on drugs when we need an unrelenting campaign for inclusion, prevention, and treatment. By permitting stigma we sanction a society that mistreats its members and thereby erodes our core human values.

While history may deliver to our societies old and poisonous views, I believe that it is the behaviors of those we do not understand or cannot countenance that perpetuate our biases and harmful ideas. For example, when people with schizophrenia appear no different from others, when they do not talk aloud to themselves or wear three ski parkas or out of their own fear instill fear in others, they become part of the flock, not painted birds. What we cannot understand, what is alien to us, evokes disquiet and triggers critical judgment. In people with substance use disorders, the behaviors many resort to to support their habit can be particularly disquieting, alienating, and even shameful. They may lie, cheat, manipulate, steal, and injure. They may prostitute themselves or sell others into the sex trade. They may lose all sight of others as they tend to the demands of their habit. They may repetitively promise to recover and start treatment only to renege and start using again.

As noted before, man takes a drink, the drink takes a drink, then the drink takes the man. F. Scott Fitzgerald is credited with a variant of this saying, but it is probably a long-standing Irish proverb. This is what I think Dr. Nora Volkow, director of the National Institute on Drug Abuse, means when she talks about drugs hijacking the brain. When the drink takes the man, it is the craving, the need to quiet withdrawal and psychic pain—not, in later stages of addiction, even the pursuit of pleasure—that drives the individual's offensive behaviors and makes him or her a pariah in his or her family and community. The terrible irony is that most of the time these people, diseased by drug addiction, know the price and are still ready to pay it.

Stigma, and discrimination, come at those with substance-use problems by three vectors. The first is how others treat them, the second is how they treat themselves, and the last is how they are treated by social institutions and services. These forces, combined, can be deadly.

There is little evidence that negative treatment of people changes them in any lasting, positive way. Yet judgment and aversion are a natural response to that which we don't like, such as lying, drunkenness, and theft. We seek to protect ourselves. We write these people off, believing they cannot be different. But the paradox is that what can help a person with a substance use disorder is just the opposite: namely, being nonjudgmental, accepting, and maintaining hope for a different future. I do not mean to suggest that anyone should put themselves in a position to be hurt or exploited; we must always put our own safety and that of loved ones first. Yet we can usually still permit an open door, a spirit of support for what is right, and a shared view of a better, more contributing future life. When we direct negative energies and feelings toward people with addictions, we drive them further into their addictive behaviors and further away from the prospect of recovery. Only one in ten people with substance use disorders gets needed and effective treatment. We help make this unholy situation happen when we stigmatize and discriminate against people with addictions. That's the first vector.

The second vector is what happens in those affected, often early, surely later, and with little chance of escape. The great actor

Samuel L. Jackson once remarked, "I guess the worst day I have had was when I had to stand up in rehab in front of my wife and daughter and say, 'Hi, my name is Sam and I am an addict.' "

Shame is more powerful than guilt in its psychological injury. Guilt is usually circumscribed and derived from violating a rule or breaking a taboo; it can be remedied by contrition or penance. Guilt can be undone, as a rule. But shame is different: it is about *the self*, how we regard ourselves in the deepest and most racking of ways. Shame is notoriously hard to undo, with few specific or effective remedies. It tends to live on and do increasing and cumulative damage as it erodes a person's self-regard. The degradation that people with addictions feel when stigmatized fuels further shame—which is a massive trigger for drug use, for blotting out what is most unbearable, self-loathing.

It has been said that the measure of a society is how it treats its poor, disadvantaged, and ill. We have problems here as well. That's the third vector. Hospitals, clinics, doctors, and even nurses eschew "addicts," don't want them cluttering their emergency rooms, medical wards, and offices. Medical professionals, ostensibly trained to diagnose and treat people with illnesses with respect, can be judgmental about addictions. The actions of some health services and professionals still reflect the long-standing belief that addiction is a moral failure, not a medical illness. Due to stigma, an addicted person's efforts to secure opioids from a doctor is not seen as a communication, a call for help, but as an exploitative move that needs to be countered with rejection.

The website of the US Department of Labor (DOL) states:

The Mental Health Parity and Addiction Equity Act of 2008 (MHPAEA) requires group health plans and health insurance issuers to ensure that financial requirements (such as co-pays, deductibles) and treatment limitations (such as visit limits) applicable to mental health or substance use disorder (MH/SUD) benefits are no more restrictive than the predominant requirements or limitations applied to substantially all medical/surgical benefits. MHPAEA supplements prior provisions under the Mental Health Parity Act of 1996 (MHPA), which required parity with respect to aggregate lifetime and annual dollar limits for mental health benefits.

Championed by former congressman Patrick J. Kennedy, with bipartisan support, this essential law was meant to counteract the discrimination against the proper detection and treatment of mental and substance use disorders rampant among medical insurers and health plans across the country. Yet it was many years before the Department of Health and Human Services (HHS) wrote the regulations needed to give the law its prescribed applications and enable enforcement. Some mental health and addiction managed-care plans sued to prevent the law from being acted upon, eventually losing, but in the meantime siphoning time and money away from care. In recent years, it has taken lawsuits to get payers to comply, as happened in New York State under Attorney General Eric Schneiderman. In 2016, President Obama ordered a task force from the Department of Labor and HHS to better overcome the barriers to this law's implementation. It costs money to treat addictions, but it costs a lot more money not to. But the money buckets are separate and incentives are perverse: money not spent on treatment saves insurance payers, but costs accrue elsewhere in social-welfare, police, and correctional programs. Legal action will be needed to help drive change, since financial and moral forces are not effectively making treatment more accessible and affordable.

Critical resources are also impacted when a person is diagnosed with an addiction. They may not be able to buy health or life insurance or only at prohibitive rates. Public housing can be denied if a person has been imprisoned, even for a nonviolent drug-possession offense. Colleges and universities tend to avoid youth with behavior problems, including addiction. And no one puts their substance use disorder on a job application unless they don't want the job.

Three vectors, three strikes, against people who are just like us, even if they are painted birds.

What might engender trust so that people with substance use problems can receive their fair share and be able to recover and serve in responsible roles, to be more included in our families and communities? There are ways.

Tony Blair, the UK prime minister from 1997 to 2007, established early in his administration a Social Exclusion Unit to implement policies to create opportunities for all to fully participate in the social and economic life of his country. This included people in poverty as well as others who, by no choice of their own, had little chance to live lives with community and contribution. This included people with mental and addictive disorders. His work has been adopted by other countries and has influenced the thinking of leaders throughout the globe.

In the United States, a number of efforts are being made against stigma.

One is Bring Change 2 Mind (BC2M), an organization founded by Glenn Close, the remarkable film, television, and stage actor, and her sister, Jessie Close, who has suffered from bipolar disorder since she was a teenager. BC2M seeks "to end the stigma and prejudice surrounding mental illness." Their efforts seek to use scientific research to alter patterns of discrimination and injustice. One such way is to improve "literacy" about behavioral conditions, including substance use disorders, and encourage people to talk openly about them. BC2M also serves as a portal to other mental health organizations that can provide additional education and treatment services. Too many people do not understand mental conditions, their causes and consequences, or where to turn for treatment. BC2M seeks to change that.

A second effort is being led by the National Council for Community Behavioral Healthcare in partnership with many other nonprofit and governmental groups. The National Council is a principal force for and training organization for Mental Health First Aid (MHFA). MHFA offers tools for any person encountering someone with a mental health or addiction problem until the crisis abates or the person receives professional help. MHFA can be especially useful to high school teachers and college educators and to clergy and first responders, as well as many others. It teaches responders how to understand what is happening, be nonjudgmental, provide support and reassurance, and encourage getting more help when needed. It is the behavioral health version of CPR. It counters the distance and aversion we all feel when we face a problem we don't understand and don't know what to do about.

I WILL LISTEN is a third, powerful anti-stigma effort created and run by the National Alliance on Mental Illness (NAMI), the largest family-led advocacy organization for mental and substance use disorders in the United States. I WILL LISTEN teaches people how to listen, how to accept, how to engage, and how to help, including directing people to where help can be obtained. I am among the large number of people NAMI has recruited to offer to listen.

BC2M, MHFA, and NAMI are important examples of how to reduce stigma. They provide information and teach skills meant to enable us all to live and work side by side, where familiarity can breed confidence and comfort as well as counter prejudice, bullying, and fear. Where the painted birds are just like us.

In closing this chapter, I want to describe what each of us, individually, can do. Laws, policies, organizations, and campaigns are vital—*and* they are augmented by the everyday actions we all can exert.

My great colleague Pat Lincourt, at a sister New York State agency (the Office of Alcoholism and Substance Abuse Services, or OASAS), has written about people with substance problems from an unapologetic and fundamentally positive perspective. Her premise is that people with addictions are indeed no different from the rest of us; if we look closely, they will defy all the stereotypes they evoke. She illustrates how these people will, if given the chance, acknowledge and take responsibility for the pain they cause others and themselves, as well as their disgrace and failed efforts to recover. They will also speak to the ambivalence a person has of using (and implicitly the purposes served by using), while highlighting the hefty price they pay for their addiction. One poignant example, from her "10 Truths People with Substance Disorder Tell," reads, "I am sorry for the pain I cause others as a result of my substance use." Lincourt describes how, though destructive behaviors cannot be excused, substance use disorders have biological and psychological underpinnings—and that people with those disorders are near-universally pained at the hurt they cause others. Her wisdom is an essential way for each of us to look past the drug and find the person who is using.

Addiction pirates the brain, but it need not pirate our humanity toward those affected. Finding ways to effectively combat stigma and discrimination can happen individually, legally, organizationally, and socially. In doing so, we do credit to our values of inclusion and tolerance, and we create some of the essential conditions and context for the successful control of drug use and abuse throughout the world.

PART THREE

CLOSING THOUGHTS

TOM'S STORY

The human heart has a want that science cannot supply.
—SIR WILLIAM OSLER

When on leave from my psychiatric residency for alternative military service, I spent two years in rural, impoverished northern Maine—in Aroostook County, about eight hours by car north of Boston and near the Canadian border. For a good part of my stay, with only eighteen months of psychiatric training, I was the only psychiatrist in this vast and hurting county.

I had three populations of patients: Anglicans, farmers mostly, some of whom were of *Mayflower* stock; French Canadians who lived on the US side of the border with Canada and did a fair amount of the forest logging; and a number of Native Americans from tribes living on reservations across the county. (I also treated members of the US Air Force and their families at Loring Air Force Base, now defunct, but that's another story.)

One day, when rounding at the community hospital where I ran ten inpatient psychiatric beds (sharing the same floor as pediatrics!), a Native family of adults arrived and wanted to see me, likely from either the Mi'kmaqs or the Maliseets, who predominated in the region. The Native Americans kept their distance from the white people, even in medical matters, so it was a surprise for a Native family to show up and ask to see the psychiatrist.

The aide brought four people into an examining room located off the shiny hospital corridor. One man looked in his fifties, while the rest—one woman and two more men—appeared to be in their twenties. One of the younger men was highly agitated, with his eyes darting around the room and full of fear. The others tried to calm him, but it didn't help much. Only by surrounding him did they keep him from bolting.

I remembered from my training to give an agitated patient plenty of room so he or she wouldn't feel cornered and slowly approached the group. The older man stepped forward and told me that his nephew Tom had been drinking heavily for months and then stopped a day or two ago. Tom wanted to quit, the man said; Tom wanted to try again at school, to be the first one in their tribe to succeed at college.

At least Tom had been drinking legal beer and spirits and not drinking denatured alcohol or inhaling Sterno (or some other poison) that would quickly destroy his brain—and with which there could be surprises in managing his withdrawal. Athletically built with long, thick, lustrous black hair, Tom was dressed in jeans, work boots, and the kind of parka that residents of the area commonly wore in winter. He looked older than his twenty-three years, and haggard. The uncle said a doctor had told Tom he had a problem with his heart, but otherwise he was "good."

When I tried to say something to Tom, he glared at me; he was grossly tremulous and sweating profusely. He was clearly in withdrawal; sweating suggests fever or worse. His nervous system was hyperaroused, with norepinephrine and cortisol being released in torrents, driving up his heart rate and blood pressure, raising body temperature and steering blood to the muscles. Under circumstances of serious threat, this is called the fight-or-flight response, evolution's kind contribution to our survival. But a body system evolved for one purpose can be rerouted, as it is in delirium tremens (DTs), a medical emergency. With the DTs, Tom's blood pressure and pulse could so elevate that his heart could not sustain its physiological demand; he could go into cardiac collapse and die, especially if he had preexisting heart disease.

I left the exam room, found the nurse on duty, and suggested that we get Tom into a single room away from everyone else. I wrote orders for detox with Librium, the choice at the time, and thiamin to prevent a rare complication of alcoholism called Wernicke's encephalopathy, in which healthy brain tissue denied this essential nutrient dies. "We need to get his vital signs and a cardiogram," I told the nurse, adding, "He doesn't look very well disposed to being touched."

About five minutes later, the nurse emerged from the exam room and walked slowly toward me. "Hello, Doctor," she said with her usual practiced formality. She had spoken with Tom's sister (the third man was his brother), and together they persuaded Tom to let the nurse take his pulse, blood pressure, and temperature. They all turned out to be too high, no surprise given what I saw clinically. But his pulse was strong and regular. In a quiet single room surrounded by his family, he took several high doses of Librium and some fluids and began to settle down. I concluded that Tom had begun the DTs with the horror, disorientation, and nervous system arousal that characterize the condition. But treatment had begun early, and he was responding. His family were never more than a few feet away from him throughout the many hours needed to stabilize him. That meant far more to him than I understood at the time.

I was witnessing a family making a lifesaving treatment possible. To get Tom to stay, at least for the first few days, I agreed that his family, however many they wanted, could share the room with him—and they did, day and night. They were his bridge to reality, his touchstone to trust, as well as protection for hospital staff should he suddenly become paranoid and strike out. The family were critical, as well, in conveying Tom's life story, not only in their words but also in their actions.

Tom's sister told me that he had been a handsome and talented adolescent with a quick mind and reflexes, one of those youths who stand out wherever they are. He was the firstborn in his family of four children. His mother died from a car accident when he was ten, leaving him in the care of her brother; Tom's father had left the family and was seldom on the reservation. The uncle was a leader on the reservation, not too heavy a drinker, and stayed close to home. Tom was a good student on a reservation where education had little value, and he became a pretty good boxer. While he would never be a contender for the Golden Gloves, he was fast and aggressive and knew how to outwit an opponent. Smart, athletic, and attractive, he stood out in a community where alcoholism, aimlessness, and unemployment were the norm among young men. Tom had enrolled in the state university, a ride south of the reservation, which provided him with free tuition and board and offered the promise of a life different from that of his friends and family. Tom was the first one to try. No other member of this reservation had ever gone away for school. That was five years before I met him.

When he quit school for the first time to come home, his family persuaded him to return. He still carried the family's hopes and pride for his achievement, and he liked the feeling of being first. But one school leave followed another. It was not the studies that got to him. Ironically, what gave him strength was also his undoing: his profound attachment to his family and community, and theirs to him, was essential to his psychic equilibrium and his capacity to succeed. Without them, he was a lost soul. Many youths can take the feeling of secure attachment with them wherever they go, but Tom's emotional security was dependent on feeling his family's presence daily and visibly—and college was hundreds of miles away.

Within a few days of arriving at the hospital, Tom was well into a controlled, medical alcohol detoxification. The DTs abated, he was able to eat, hold down food, and sleep, though fitfully. It was weeks before Tom would be ready to leave the hospital, using the time to rebuild his health and regain some of his confidence and hope for the future. I was in no rush to discharge him, and he and his family had more or less set up camp there anyway. As the DTs passed and his acute withdrawal was complete, further evaluation done on his heart revealed evidence of some enlargement. It didn't need medical treatment, but would heal itself if he stayed away from alcohol and its cardiac toxicity. I came to see the charm and intelligence that had won him so many supporters and opportunities. I began to think he could return to school once again. But he could not and would not. He seemed to know that.

When he was due for discharge from the hospital, I offered to see him as an outpatient in one of my clinics. I had patients throughout the county and rode a circuit regularly from the southern town of Houlton to various French border towns such as Fort Kent and Madawaska. Mostly I saw people in consultation or to prescribe medications, working with psychologists and social workers who provided the ongoing therapy. This type of team care has only become more necessary to meet the needs of people with substance use and mental disorders in this country, especially in rural and underserved communities.

Tom came to see me four or five times as an outpatient in the year that followed. He would make an appointment and then, usually, either not show up or call to cancel. When he came, it was always with family. I tried to understand what he wanted and what stood in his way, a practical version of therapy, but in retrospect I think I had an inadequate understanding of his dilemma. I did not fully appreciate how family and community were his psychological oxygen, and that he could not emotionally breathe without them. I never visited him on the reservation, which I regret. I did not understand that when he did not come to me, I needed to go to him. I did not work with him and his family in a way that recognized that they were one entity, one living organism, which could not bear separation. I had a lot to learn—not that I'm now finished.

Over the year or so I was his doctor, Tom would work some, stay sober, and then start drinking again. When he was drinking, he was most at ease with himself and his community. He was part of them. He was safe. I see that now. He did not have to try to scale the emotional wall of guilt and disloyalty he felt in leaving, no matter how noble or idealized the pursuit seemed to be to his family and friends. Nor did he have to feel the insecure attachment, the separation anxiety that emerged when he was apart from his family and community. By staying and living the life of the reservation, with its intensely intertwined families and the bonding that drinking among the men provided, he could satisfy his needs, every day, even at what would be so great a cost.

Tom was years into and dependent on a mind-numbing and physically addictive substance before he came for care. I wonder what might have been different had his school, his family, and his community been able to foster early on a secure sense of attachment and the inner capacity to stand on his own while still being fully connected to those he loved. His set, or underlying psychic nature or personality, had been shaped by trauma and adversity and was built on dependent, not independent, attachments. Maybe, I thought back then, he could achieve the independence he needed to successfully leave his family (and his addiction) and become his own man. But I know now that his community, his context or setting, was such that drinking was normative and exit to a different life, apart, was improbable.

The last time I saw Tom, he was drinking again. He told me he had begun a medication for his heart, for an arrhythmia, or irregular heartbeat, that he had developed. He said, "The family doctor who came to the reservation said my heart had problems from the drinking. . . . He said my heart muscle had gone kind of soft. I'm going to get sober again. . . . I can do it."

After my two years of service, in 1974 I left Aroostook County to resume my residency. I had a bad sense about what would befall Tom.

Some years later I revisited northern Maine, at that glorious time in early July when all the potato fields are in blossom, looking like endless white and pink blankets warming the earth as they stretch to the blue horizon. I went to see my friends at the mental health center. They told me about Tom. He had died about a year after I left of a fatal arrhythmia caused by myocarditis, a cardiac complication of alcoholism. One day when drinking, he dropped to the ground, dead, while walking around the reservation.

Tom's story comes back to me now as I write this book. He was my first extended and profound immersion into substance use, abuse, and disorder. To set and setting. To secure and insecure attachments. To trauma too, namely for Tom's losing his mother at age ten.

Back then, there was AA, but not for Native Americans. Back then there was no SBIRT, screening for problem drinking and drug use, especially in adolescents, so that early intervention might be possible. Back then there was no MAT, medication-assisted treatment; he would have been a candidate for long-acting naltrexone (Vivitrol) had it existed. He had the support of his family, but that had its paradoxical side because he could not pursue a life away, a life of his own. There were no relapse prevention groups or CBT to help him regulate his impulses and self-destructive behaviors.

My memory of Tom, his people, a world of unattainable opportunities, leaves me pained and empty. It also reminds me about how much we have learned about more successfully working with people with addictions. And it gives me the drive to keep trying to make a difference in the lives of people with substance use disorders, their families, and their communities.

APPENDIX

A Brief History of Opioid
Use and Abuse in America

Medical historians of addiction like to consider three, maybe four, eras of drug use in America. But a closer look reveals five eras, extending from this country's earliest days through the opioid epidemic presently seizing the United States.

The historiography of addiction points to an age-old debate: Does addiction derive from weak character, calling for criminalization, regulation, and stigma, as well as recovery approaches built on the twentieth-century 12-step model, a spiritual path meant to reclaim the addict's soul? Or is it a medical problem, undeserving of stigma and discrimination, which calls for humane prevention and treatment? These are the two competing visions, bad versus ill, that have done battle in this country for over two hundred years—and persist today, despite an abundance of evidence for the latter.

A first era, often little noted, was depicted in the scandalous and popular *Confessions of an English Opium-Eater* by Thomas De Quincey, published in 1821. This paean to laudanum (opium dissolved in alcohol and imbibed) tells the story of De Quincey's first use of opium, considered of little risk, to relieve his joint pains. This pattern is eerily similar to that of the last twenty years of opioid use in America, when prescription pain pills provided by doctors spurred on by pharmaceutical advertisements and assurances of a low risk of addiction were instrumental in fostering the epidemic we now have. De Quincey wrote, "Happiness might now be bought for a penny . . . portable ecstasies might be had corked up in a pint bottle."

De Quincey wasn't the only regular user of laudanum at that time. Laudanum and "black drop" opium, two variants of extracts from the poppy plant, were easily accessible from the beginning of the nineteenth century. Laudanum, which contained alcohol, and black drop, which did not, were available in a host of patent medications as well as by prescription. They provided calming and sedating effects and were used to treat many conditions, from gastrointestinal and other physical illnesses to emotional problems. The drugs were inexpensive, reportedly had limited potential for abuse, and were regarded as having little effect on a person's functioning. Doctors generally thought the risk of dependence was small and, when it existed, was more likely among the lower socioeconomic classes. The medicinal use of these opioids and the criminal justice system did not interact. Since the benefits of laudanum and opium were considered to exceed the risks, they were commonly employed.

Their popularity was in part because doctors in this country (and abroad) had but a limited number of interventions for the multitude of patient problems they encountered: at the time, "the therapeutic arsenal was a trinity of emetics, purgatives and bloodletting (including the use of leeches)." A panacea as powerful as opium was sure to be widely adopted and was even termed "God's Own Medicine." Broadly utilized, it was reportedly a popular treatment for "female problems" among middle-class white women who suffered pain and other conditions more "nervous" in nature, predominantly neurasthenia (a syndrome of unexplained etiology characterized by fatigue, headaches, and irritability).

The second era has gained far more attention given the many developments in drug use and abuse between the mid-1800s and the turn of the twentieth century. In 1852, Scottish physician Alexander Wood and French physician Charles Pravaz independently and more or less simultaneously introduced the hypodermic (literally, "under the skin") syringe to hasten the delivery of drugs. Wood was the first, in 1853, to inject a patient with morphine, which revolutionized medicine and drug addiction. The first known death from morphine overdose was Wood's wife, who had used the drug to excess.

The Civil War in the United States produced a tragic abundance of injured and disabled soldiers suffering physical and psychic pain, many of whom became dependent on opioids. Their addiction was called soldier's disease. Estimates are that four hundred thousand were addicted by the war's end in 1865 from the liberal use of opium pills and morphine injections, and morphine use then spread from veterans to many people suffering chronic pain. By the end of the nineteenth century, the use of intramuscular morphine in America was reportedly considerably greater than in other developed Western countries, including in Europe, where war wounds were no less present.

In a landmark event in the history of opioids, in 1898 Bayer Pharmaceuticals, a German corporation, developed and introduced heroin, initially as a cough medicine as well as for controlling menstrual pain. The German word for this drug was *heroisch*, meaning powerful, and it was. In America that same year, a New York physician at Mt. Sinai Hospital championed the use of heroin and published in the *New York Medical Journal* an article titled "Treatment of Coughs with Heroin."

Thus, by the end of the nineteenth century, opioids, especially morphine and heroin, had achieved widespread medical use. Their ingestion would only escalate in the coming decades.

During the latter part of the nineteenth century, as mentioned earlier in this book, the use of opium was also common among Chinese immigrants. It provided analgesia and psychic relief for immigrants pressed into hard labor in a foreign land building its railroads.

Concerns about the abuse of opium abroad, especially in China, helped foster the beginnings of the Temperance Movement in this country. Social pressures led initially to reductions in consumption of opium, and doctors became more aware of the risks of dependence from their liberal prescribing practices. As the century came to a close, an attitudinal shift began, away from appreciating opioids' medicinal use and toward seeing their use as a moral failing, worthy of criminal justice approaches to their control. So began the infamous War on Drugs, though it was not called that until nearly a century later.

There was no evidence that the use of opioids destroyed body tissue or organs. So popular opinion determined that the social and psychological deterioration seen in those dependent on opioids was not due to their physical effects on the brain or other parts of the anatomy. Users became dependent, the thinking went, because they had weak characters that bent to the drug.

By 1900 an estimated quarter million people in this country were addicted to opioids. Morphine clinics sprang up where users could go daily for an intramuscular injection, but social attitudes were becoming more intolerant. Alcoholism, syphilis infection, and opioid dependence were soon considered vices that occurred principally among poor people of the lower classes. These attitudinal shifts made medicinal use of opioids unappealing and set the stage for the regulation of the drugs that followed in the twentieth century. But at that time, only modest tariffs limited the importation of opium, and patent medicines containing opium (and cocaine) were still common. Efforts by states to limit their use were not effective, though in some states a physician's prescription became necessary to buy the medicines.

Enter the third era, which commenced with the first half of the twentieth century, when shifting attitudes toward opioid use took greater hold. Epitomizing this shift, in 1903, Dr. George Pettey, an addiction specialist, vocalized a growing opinion about the depravity of addiction, calling it "another curse."

A series of federal regulations, beginning with the Pure Food and Drug Act of 1906, were bellwethers for the changing national outlook on drugs and drug dependence. This federal legislation represented an early regulatory effort at consumer protection and also made illegal importing opium that could be smoked.

The Pure Food and Drug Act paved the way for the creation of the Food and Drug Administration (FDA), with its more public-health vision that aimed to protect and promote the well-being of the citizens of this country. On the further authority of the Pure Food and Drug Act, in 1909 the importation of opium for smoking was more substantively prohibited. But like today, the use, abuse, and dependence upon opium (and its natural and synthetic variants, called the opioids) in America did not wane despite the illegality of its importation.

A few years later, the Harrison Narcotics Tax Act of 1914 ushered in a federal system for regulating physician prescribing, drug manufacturing, and pharmacy distribution. The State Department drove its passage, aiming to curtail the growth of the poppy plant (the source of opium and its natural derivatives) in China and build lucrative trade agreements with that vastly populated country.

With the passage of this act, the landscape for drugs became very different in America. The act made illegal the prescription of morphine for the treatment or ongoing maintenance of addiction. It criminalized drug addiction and its medical care. It pushed opium- and heroin-dependent individuals toward illegal sources of drugs, fostering crime for its importation and distribution, as well as a means for individuals to obtain the money needed to pay for their substance addiction. In addition, over three thousand physicians were jailed for refusing to stop prescribing opioids for their patients, further entangling the criminal justice system with drug use.

Of course, this criminal justice approach to drug use and abuse was ineffective in reducing the use and abuse of opioids, just as it has been in more recent times.

Heroin use reportedly reached epidemic levels of abuse in the years after World War I, as it did after both World War II and the Vietnam War, a harbinger of the fourth era of drugs in America. Because US regulations prohibited heroin's use, it was distributed through illegal markets.

Yet, medical professionals still considered the risk of heroin dependence to be low; use of the drug was regarded as evidence of immoral character, prevalent among criminals. Nevertheless, heroin's popularity continued to climb. The typical person dependent on heroin at that time was white, city dwelling, and poor; New York City was an epicenter of activity, remaining so until recent years when heroin (and opioid) use has spread widely to Middle American towns and cities. By the 1920s, thanks to the Harrison Act, drug-dependent people *and* doctors were filling the cells of the federal penitentiary at Leavenworth, Kansas.

We now arrive at the fourth era of opioids in America, the years after World War II until the end of the millennium.

By the decades after World War II, heroin had become the principal opioid of abuse in this country. Annual estimates of its use became available from the Monitoring the Future national survey beginning in 1975, and then from the National Survey on Drug Use and Health (NSDUH), which eclipsed the earlier survey by the early 1990s. The use of heroin was also a part of the culture of the 1960s, where drug experimentation among youth was not confined to cannabis and psychedelic drugs. One report indicated a tenfold increase in heroin users from 1960 to 1970, involving baby boomers and suburban dwellers. If we are looking for evidence that control strategies and criminalization of drug users do not work, the mid-twentieth century gives us plenty.

Yet there was also the renaissance of a medical understanding of opioids, drug dependence, and the proper care of drug users. The concept of addiction as a disease began to gain some traction in the minds of American policy makers. In the 1960s, at the Rockefeller Institute in New York (now called Rockefeller University), Drs. Vincent Dole and Marie Nyswander began to advance the use of methadone, a synthetic drug that worked on the same brain receptors as morphine and heroin. This potent opioid was to be taken orally, like many of the prescription opioid drugs produced today. (Though methadone can be administered intramuscularly as well, that was not what the two doctors sought to introduce.)

Their success in providing methadone as a maintenance treatment for heroin addiction was groundbreaking. Methadone resulted, especially, in reductions in criminal behaviors among people addicted to opioids because this drug could occupy the same brain reward receptors as heroin—without the risk that patients might use syringes to get high or commit crimes to pay for drugs. In 1972, methadone was made legal, and the FDA issued regulations for its use. It remains federally regulated to this day and has helped countless drug-dependent individuals have lives of greater safety, both for them and their communities. But its use has always been limited, to only a fraction of those estimated to be dependent on opioids over the ensuing decades. In addition, its appeal among heroin- and opioid-dependent people has not been high. The daily visits to clinics to receive the liquid drug, the observed administration of the medication, urine analyses for other drugs, and the frequently required psychological services were often not welcomed by people affected by the disease of drug addiction. Moreover, AA and later NA were vocally opposed to the use of one drug of potential abuse to treat another. Communities, as well, did not like methadone clinics in their neighborhoods because of the crime zones they could create.

No history of drug use in America is complete without mention of President Richard Nixon's War on Drugs. Nixon was the first to use the metaphor of the War on Drugs, and his strategy was to combine criminalizing drug use in this country with military intervention in other countries. Many considered Nixon's approach an effort to punish people of color and hippies, central to his Southern strategy to win reelection; he couldn't have cared less about drug dependence in America. This view was later supported by John Ehrlichman, Nixon's domestic-policy chief, who said as much in an interview a couple of decades later.

In 1973, the Drug Enforcement Administration (DEA) was launched to further strengthen efforts to control drug use and distribution in America. A review of its history suggests that for many years it was an ineffective agency known for internal battles more than battling drug problems in this country.

The casualties of Nixon's "war," however, have been enormous, and no evidence of its benefits has been demonstrated by any responsible government, including our own. Since President Nixon declared this war, the incarceration rate in the United States has increased by over 400 percent and is now the highest in the world. Aided and abetted by President and Mrs. Ronald Reagan, the war continued. By 1994, this war had led to a million Americans arrested *each year* for drugs, with about one in four arrests for marijuana possession; more recently marijuana has been the charge in half of the arrests in this country.

Another momentous period before 2000 was the Vietnam War years. Not only did it produce great domestic turmoil, but it also gave legions of American soldiers immediate access to high-potency heroin that might help them bear the conditions (and stigma) of an unpopular war. While far fewer veterans persisted in their addiction when they came home, an estimated 12 percent did, adding to its prevalence in this country.

Two enormous, interacting events in the 1990s set the stage for the fifth era, the one in which we currently live.

First, Purdue Pharmaceuticals, the maker of OxyContin, drew upon scientifically flimsy evidence to declare that the use of its branded opioid carried essentially no risk of addiction. A 1980 report in the *New England Journal of Medicine* by Dr. Jane Porter asserted that of twenty-two hundred people on Oxy-Contin, a mere four became addicted. This spurious research was amplified in 1986 by a letter in the *Journal of Pain* by Dr. Russell Portenoy, a prominent pain specialist, stating that only four of twenty-four people treated with OxyContin became addicted. These reports became the basis of a vast marketing campaign by Purdue that resulted in, as just one example, the delivery of 780 million (!) opioid pain pills to West Virginia— one of the epicenters of the opioid epidemic in this century. Purdue later settled a suit for misrepresenting their product and paid over $600 million, which I imagine is a small fraction of their profits.

The other event in the busy 1990s accelerating the problems of opioid use and abuse was a decision by the American Pain Society to call pain the fifth vital sign, joining blood pressure, pulse, respiration, and temperature as the essential measurements doctors need to perform upon seeing every patient. A simple pain scale, 1–10, would do, and there would be hospital-accreditation and medical-license implications for failure to assess a person's level of pain. In all fairness, pain had likely been both under- and overtreated before the fifth vital sign was introduced. But once it was in place, doctors had endless evidence, from required reporting forms, concerning patient pain—and the handiest and fastest way to respond was to write a prescription for an opioid pain pill.

Today, we are now well into the fifth era in the history of opioids in America, and by far the deadliest.

Heroin use in the United States has slowly but steadily risen since 2002. Overdose deaths, as well, have been on an unceasing and rapid rise since 2002, attributable (until very recently) to the use of opioid pain pills. In the past few years, the increase, despite reductions in opioid pain pill prescriptions, has been the result of the resurgence in the use of heroin, now often cut with the far more lethal drug fentanyl. The CDC has recently become active in tracking the opioid epidemic in America.

The recent, marked increases in heroin use and heroin use disorder in this country have been greater among whites than among black or Hispanic people. The growth in heroin use can be attributed, in part, to a progression from taking opioid prescription pills, prescribed more readily to white people than people of color by doctors, to snorting and finally injecting heroin when supplies of pills from doctors become difficult to access and the street costs too great for the user. In effect, the rebound in heroin use is now a "solution" for those dependent on prescription opioid pills who need a cheaper and readier source of drugs.

The greater availability of heroin, as well as its increased potency and lower prices, appear related to increased activity among cartels and other criminal distributors. Our failed policies and practices have been good for business for the bad guys.

Heroin use has increased more among men than women in this period. This has been understood, in part, as a result of reductions in manufacturing and the joblessness this creates, chronic pain from years of physical labor, and few prospects for middle-aged men, and for their children.

The most chilling evidence of increasing drug use and abuse in America is the extraordinary rise in prescriptions of opioid pain pills in the last fifteen years (despite recent modest reductions in their numbers in some states). The phenomenal quantity of individual prescriptions written and the total pills prescribed speaks to the explosion of use, abuse, and dependence on them that has swept this country. Opioid prescriptions in 2010 were four times what they were in 1999, commensurate with a fourfold increase in overdose deaths from 1988 to 2008. Overdose deaths, as noted, were principally from opioid prescription medications, though heroin (and fentanyl) have begun to gain hegemony.

The opioid addiction epidemic now ravaging this country exceeds dependency on any other substance, including alcohol, marijuana, and cocaine.

An important innovation in this fifth era is a new medical treatment of opioid dependence, which has not been widely adopted despite its strong promise. In 2002, introduced by federal legislation called DATA 2000, an office-based prescription treatment for opioid dependence became legal and available in the United States. The medication is buprenorphine, an opioid taken sublingually (and more recently in other preparations) that occupies the same brain receptors as do heroin, morphine, and prescription opioids. The hope was that because a month's supply could be prescribed by a physician who took a course and registered with the Drug Enforcement Administration, this agent would help stem the tide of growing opioid dependence in America. But its prescription has been slow—first with doctors being limited to treating a maximum of only 30 patients (later 100, and now with special permission 275), limited insurance coverage and payment, required training (the only drug in America requiring a course and a special DEA license designation), and stigma among the medical community regarding people with substance use disorders. The gap remains too great: many more people can benefit from buprenorphine than currently do.

WHAT'S AHEAD?

What can be done to understand and respond better to our country's opioid epidemic? And to the use of, abuse of, and dependence on other common drugs such as alcohol, cocaine, crystal meth, stimulant pills, tranquilizers, sedatives, and marijuana?

The answers do not lie in an ongoing attachment and investment in the criminalization of drug use and abuse. The answers do not lie in exhorting people to stop, young and not so young. The answers are public-health in nature: prevention, early intervention, effective and comprehensive treatment programs, and a cultural shift toward understanding not just the neuroscience of addiction but also the psychological and social dimensions central to the commencement and continuation of addictive behaviors.

Today we are witnessing a high point of drug use that exceeds that in all prior eras, and this is especially true of opioid use. Deaths from overdoses from opioid prescription medications have far exceeded those from heroin for over fifteen years, though heroin overdoses have escalated considerably in recent years. As previously noted, by 2013, opioid sales and dependence had exceeded dependence on either alcohol, cocaine, and marijuana, and deaths from opioids now exceed those from gunshot wounds and motor vehicle accidents, combined.

Yet for all the human and social ravages opioid and other addictive drugs have wrought, no substantive relief seems in sight, especially if this country continues to pursue puritanical, punitive, and political solutions rather than those drawn from science and public-health practices.

Solutions, many described in this book, are plentiful and effective. Their adoption and widespread dissemination is up to us.

BOOKS THAT
MAY BE OF INTEREST

Blackburn, Elizabeth, and Elissa Epel. *The Telomere Effect*. New York: Grand Central Publishing, 2017.

Booth, Martin. *Opium: A History*. New York: St. Martin's Griffin, 1996.

Bradley, Elizabeth H., and Lauren A. Taylor. *The American Health Care Paradox*. New York: Public Affairs/Perseus, 2013.

Branson, Richard, ed. *Ending the War on Drugs*. London: Virgin Books, 2016.

Brown, Richard, Patricia Gerbarg, and Philip Muskin. *Complementary and Integrative Treatments in Psychiatric Practice*. Arlington, VA: American Psychiatric Association Publishing, 2017.

———. *How to Use Herbs, Nutrients, and Yoga in Mental Health Care*. New York: W. W. Norton, 2012 (paperback).

Chasin, Alexandra. *Assassin of Youth: A Kaleidoscopic History of Harry J. Anslinger's War on Drugs*. Chicago: University of Chicago Press, 2016.

Christensen, Clayton M. *The Innovator's Dilemma*. New York: HarperBusiness, 2000.

Compton, Michael T., ed. *Marijuana and Mental Health*. Arlington, VA: American Psychiatric Association Publishing, 2016.

Compton, Michael T., and Ruth S. Shim, eds. *The Social Determinants of Mental Health*. Arlington, VA: American Psychiatric Association Publishing, 2015.

De Quincey, Thomas. *Confessions of an English Opium-Eater.* London: Crescent Press, 1950.

Doidge, Norman. *The Brain's Way of Healing.* New York: Penguin, 2015.

Foote, Jeffrey, Carrie Wilkins, and Nicole Kosanke, with Stephanie Higgs. *Beyond Addiction: How Science and Kindness Help People Change.* New York: Scribner, 2014.

Hari, Johann. *Chasing the Scream.* New York: Bloomsbury, 2015.

Hart, Carl. *High Price.* New York: Harper Perennial, 2014.

Jones, Jill. *Hep-Cats, Narcs, and Pipe Dreams: A History of America's Romance with Illegal Drugs.* New York: Scribner, 1996.

Karch, Steven B. *A Brief History of Cocaine.* 2nd ed. Boca Raton, FL: Taylor & Francis, 2006.

Kennedy, Patrick J., and Stephen Fried. *A Common Struggle.* New York: Blue Rider Press, 2015.

Leary, Timothy, Ralph Metzner, and Richard Alpert. *The Psychedelic Experience: A Manual Based on* The Tibetan Book of the Dead. New York: Citadel Press, 1992.

Levounis, Petros, Erin Zerbo, and Rashi Aggarwal, eds. *The Pocket Guide to Addiction Assessment and Treatment.* Arlington, VA: American Psychiatric Association Publishing, 2016.

Lewis-Fernández, R., N. K. Aggarwal, L. Hinton, D. E. Hinton, and L. J. Kirmayer, eds. *DSM-5 Handbook on the Cultural Formulation Interview.* Arlington, VA: American Psychiatric Association Publishing, 2016.

Marlatt, G. Alan, and D. M. Donovan, eds. *Relapse Prevention: Maintenance Strategies in the Treatment of Addictive Behaviors.* 2nd ed. New York: Guilford, 2005.

Maté, Gabor. *In the Realm of Hungry Ghosts.* Berkeley, CA: North Atlantic Books, 2008.

Milkman, Harvey B., and Stanley Sunderwirth. *Craving for Ecstasy*. San Francisco: Jossey-Bass, 1998.

Miller, William, and Stephen Rollnick. *Motivational Interviewing: Helping People Change*. 3rd ed. New York: Guilford, 2013.

Mukherjee, Siddhartha. *The Gene*. New York: Scribner, 2016.

Musto, David F. *The American Disease: Origins of Narcotic Controls*. New Haven, CT: Yale University Press, 1973.

———. *Drugs in America*. New York: New York University Press, 2002.

Pollan, Michael. *The Botany of Desire*. New York: Random House, 2002.

Prochaska, James O., and Janice M. Prochaska. *Changing to Thrive*. Center City, MN: Hazelden Publishing, 2016.

Quinones, Sam. *Dream Land*. New York: Bloomsbury, 2015.

Ramsey, Drew. *Eat Complete*. New York: Harper Wave, 2016.

Sacks, Oliver. *On the Move: A Life*. New York: Knopf, 2015.

Sederer, Lloyd I. *The Family Guide to Mental Health Care*. New York: W. W. Norton, 2013.

———. *Improving Mental Health: Four Secrets in Plain Sight*. Arlington, VA: American Psychiatric Association Publishing, 2017.

Springsteen, Bruce. *Born to Run*. New York: Simon & Schuster, 2016.

Sweet, Victoria. *God's Hotel*. New York: Riverhead Books, 2012.

Szasz, Thomas. *Ceremonial Chemistry*. Garden City, NY: Anchor Press/Doubleday, 1974.

Wainwright, Thomas. *Narconomics*. New York: Public Affairs, 2016.

Waldman, Ayelet. *A Really Good Day*. New York: Grand Central Publishing, 2017.

Wanberg, Kenneth W., and Harvey B. Milkman. *Criminal Conduct and Substance Abuse Treatment: Strategies for Self-Improvement and Change: The Provider's Guide.* 2nd ed. Thousand Oaks, CA: Sage Publications, 2008.

Weil, Andrew. *The Natural Mind.* Boston: Houghton Mifflin, 2004.

White, William. *Slaying the Dragon: The History of Addiction Treatment and Recovery in America.* Bloomington, IL: Chestnut Health Systems, 1998.

Zinberg, Norman E. *Drug, Set, and Setting.* New Haven, CT: Yale University Press, 1984.

NOTES

AUTHOR'S NOTE

x   *Sales of prescription opioids in the United States:* Bertha K. Madras, "The Surge of Opioid Use, Addiction, and Overdoses: Responsibility and Response of the US Health Care System," *JAMA Psychiatry*, March 29, 2017; and Silvia S. Martins et al., "Changes in US Lifetime Heroin Use and Heroin Use Disorder Prevalence from the 2001–2002 to 2012–2013 National Epidemiologic Survey on Alcohol and Related Conditions," *JAMA Psychiatry*, March 29, 2017.

x   *The greatest increases in recent years:* Madras, "Surge of Opioid Use"; and Martins et al., "Changes in US Lifetime Heroin Use."

x   *Drug overdose deaths today exceed:* https://mises.org/blog/dea-releases -new-drug-overdose-death-figures-guns-safer-prescription-drugs; and http://www.cnsnews.com/news/article/susan-jones/dea-drug -overdoses-kill-more-americans-car-crashes-or-firearms.

x   *Over 60 percent of these avoidable deaths:* https://www.cdc.gov/media /releases/2013/p0220_drug_overdose_deaths.html.

x   *Overdose deaths from this and related opioids tripled:* From the director of the National Institute on Drug Addiction, Nora Volkow, https:// www.cdc.gov/drugoverdose/.

xi   *Cardinal Health allegedly shipped 241 million opioid pills:* From the National Conference of State Legislatures (NCSL), "American Epidemic: Overdosed on Opioids," April 1, 2016, http://www.globaldrug policy.org/Issues/Vol%2011%20Issue%201/Commentary/The%20 Worst%20Drug%20Epidemic%20in%20US%20History.pdf.

xi   *Estimates are that four out of five:* https://www.drugabuse.gov/publica tions/research-reports/relationship-between-prescription-drug-heroin -abuse/prescription-opioid-use-risk-factor-heroin-use; and http://www .nejm.org/doi/full/10.1056/NEJMra1508490#t=article.

NOTES

xi *In 2012 alone, 259 million opioid prescriptions:* https://www.cdc.gov
/vitalsigns/opioid-prescribing/.

xi *The world economies nowadays annually spend:* Richard Branson, ed.,
Ending the War on Drugs (London Virgin Books, 2016).

INTRODUCTION

5 *Buprenorphine had just been federally approved:* NYC Department
of Health and Mental Hygiene, https://www1.nyc.gov/assets/doh
/downloads/pdf/chi/chi-34-1.pdf.

CHAPTER 1: TEN THINGS THAT MATTER

11 *"That humanity at large":* Aldous Huxley, *The Doors of Perception*
(New York: Perennial Library, 1970), 62–63.

11 *"to understand how and why":* Norman Zinberg, *Drug, Set, and Setting*
(New Haven: Yale University Press, 1984), vii.

12 *One remarkable story comes to mind:* Jill Jones, *Hep-Cats, Narcs, and
Pipe Dreams: A History of America's Romance with Illegal Drug*s (New
York: Scribner 1996); and Abigail Zuger, "Traveling a Primeval Med-
ical Landscape," *News York Times*, April 26, 2010.

14 *Teens who smoke cigarettes by the time:* US Department of Health
and Human Services, Substance Abuse and Mental Health Services
Administration, Center for Behavioral Health Statistics and Qual-
ity, *National Survey on Drug Use and Health*, 2014, ICPSR36361-v1
(Ann Arbor, MI: Inter-university Consortium for Political and Social
Research [distributor], March 22, 2016), http://doi.org/10.3886
/ICPSR36361.v1.

15 *the successor agency to the former Department of Prohibition:* Alexandra
Chasin, *Assassin of Youth: A Kaleidoscopic History of Harry J. Ansling-
er's War on Drugs* (Chicago: University of Chicago Press, 2016); and
Johann Hari, *Chasing the Scream* (New York: Bloomsbury, 2015).

16 *Her psychic pain became the driver:* Zinberg, *Drug, Set, and Setting*.

16 *first, personality, the preexisting character of a person:* Ibid.

17 *Moreover, attention focused on the indicia:* N. E. Zinberg, "Heroin Use in
Vietnam and the US," *Archives of General Psychiatry* 26 (1972): 486–88.

19 *Many were seeking a means to "make time go away":* Ibid.

19 *Moreover, we know today that up to 30 percent:* Rand Corporation, https://www.rand.org/health/projects/veterans.html.

19 *declared tobacco to have a substantially greater risk:* Scientific Committee on Emerging and Newly Identified Health Risks (SCENIHR), *Addictiveness and Attractiveness of Tobacco Additives,* 2010.

19 *Cocaine snorted is less addictive:* Ibid.

26 *Cannabidiol has been sold as a dietary supplement:* C. D. Schubart et al., "Cannabis with High Cannabidiol Content Is Associated with Fewer Psychotic Experiences," *Schizophrenia Research,* May 2011.

26 *Lennox-Gastaut syndrome, another form of severe epilepsy:* American *Academy of Neurology News,* April 21, 2017.

26 *an alternative to the common antipsychotics:* Schubart et al., "Cannabis with High Cannabidiol Content."

26 *in his popular book* The Natural Mind*:* Andrew Weil, *The Natural Mind* (Boston: Houghton Mifflin, 2004), 42.

27 *nicotine patches can control cravings:* Rates of quitting tobacco with nicotine replacement are not high: http://www.tobaccofree.org/quitting.

27 *Yet this mode of treatment appears to be effective:* https://www.ncbi.nlm.nih.gov/pubmedhealth/PMH0010505/.

CHAPTER 2: DIMENSIONS OF CHARACTER

36 *a set of what are called* ego defenses*:* See also Anna Freud, *The Ego and the Mechanisms of Defence* (Karnac Books, first published in 1936), as well as https://psychcentral.com/lib/15-common-defense-mechanisms/.

CHAPTER 3: FAIL FIRST

44 *though that does not mean offensive delays:* K. Rahul, R. K. Nayak, and S. D. Pearson, "The Ethics of 'Fail First': Guidelines and Practical Scenarios for Step Therapy Coverage Policies," *Health Affairs* 33 (October 2014): 101779–85.

44 *President Lyndon Johnson's "all-out war on human poverty":* http://prde.upress.virginia.edu/content/WarOnPoverty.

45 *making the war fundamentally racist:* David F. Musto, *Drugs in America* (New York: New York University Press, 2002).

45 *Did we know we were lying:* http://harpers.org/archive/2016/04/legalize-it-all/.

46 *nonviolent drug law offenses went:* https://www.brennancenter.org/publication/how-many-americans-are-unnecessarily-incarcerated.

47 *more vigorous law enforcement and drug interdiction:* http://content.time.com/time/magazine/article/0,9171,962371-1,00.html.

47 *Public education, prevention, and rehabilitation:* https://web.stanford.edu/class/e297c/poverty_prejudice/paradox/htele.html.

47 *We know, as well, that two-thirds:* Vera Center, https://www.vera.org/.

47 *Among inmates, suicide is now the leading:* https://www.brennancenter.org/publication/how-many-americans-are-unnecessarily-incarcerated.

47 *It took until 2009 to start to move:* http://www.huffingtonpost.com/lloyd-i-sederer-md/addiction-treatment-_b_1665302.html.

48 *crop control, border interdiction, and state:* https://www.vera.org/.

48 *Our former president also commuted the sentences:* https://www.brennancenter.org/publication/how-many-americans-are-unnecessarily-incarcerated.

48 *creative members of Fictionless:* http://www.fictionless.com/.

48 *people whose punishment did not fit the crime:* http://www.huffingtonpost.com/lloyd-i-sederer-md/addiction-treatment-_b_1665302.html.

50 *Yet, the principal strategies for drug control:* http://www.cnn.com/2016/02/15/world/mexico-drug-graphics/.

51 *Addiction is "self-induced changes":* http://www.huffingtonpost.com/lloyd-i-sederer-md/addiction-treatment-_b_1665302.html.

52 *Homicides in Mexico peaked at almost twenty-three thousand:* http://www.cnn.com/2016/02/15/world/mexico-drug-graphics/.

53 *Estimates are that today over 1 million lives:* https://www.media.volvocars.com/uk/en-gb/media/pressreleases/20505.

56 *Motivation to change can come from:* W. R. Miller and S. Rollnick, *Motivational Interviewing: Preparing People for Change*, 3rd ed. (New York: Guilford, 2013).

CHAPTER 4: AN OUNCE OR A TON?

60 *producing a 5,500 percent return on investment:* J. Lightwood and S. A. Glantz, "The Effect of the California Tobacco Control Program on Smoking Prevalence, Cigarette Consumption, and Healthcare Costs: 1989–2008," *PLoS ONE* 8, no. 2 (2013): e47145.

60 *serve youth showing indicia of early behavioral:* IOM (Institute of Medicine), *Reducing Risks for Mental Disorders: Frontiers for Preventive Intervention Research* (Washington, DC: National Academy Press, 1994).

62 *ACEs occur before a child reaches:* "Relationship Between Multiple Forms of Childhood Maltreatment and Adult Mental Health in Community Respondents," *American Journal of Psychiatry*, September 2003, doi:10.1176/appi.ajp.160.8.1453.

64 *Diseases and disorders mount, limiting functioning:* J. P. Shonkoff et al., "The Lifelong Effects of Early Childhood Adversity and Toxic Stress," *Pediatrics* 129, no. 1 (January 2012): e232–e246, PMID:22201156; and K. M. Scott et al., "Association of Childhood Adversities and Early-Onset Mental Disorders with Adult-Onset Chronic Physical Conditions," *Archives of General Psychiatry* 68 (August 2011).

64 *Frederick Douglass said:* http://www.goodreads.com/quotes/28899 -it-is-easier-to-build-strong-children-than-to-repair.

66 *A second example is the enduring program Big Brothers Big Sisters:* http:// www.bbbs.org/2017/01/big-impacts-power-woman-empowers-little/.

67 *We have alternatives, but so far their adoption:* K. W. Griffin and G. J. Botvin, "Evidence-Based Interventions for Preventing Substance Use Disorders in Adolescents," *Child and Adolescent Psychiatric Clinics of North America* 19, no. 3 (July 2010): 505–26, doi:10.1016/j .chc.2010.03.005. A wonderfully arousing TEDMED Talk on ACEs, by Dr. Nadine Burke Harris, is at https://www.ted.com/talks/nadine _burke_harris_how_childhood_trauma_affects_health_across_a _lifetime?language=en.

68 *LST shows sustained effects with preventing:* Institute of Medicine, *Unleashing the Power of Prevention*, 2015.

68 *There is considerable flexibility in where and when:* http://www .strengtheningfamiliesprogram.org/.

68 *The time is right, as well, for introducing:* http://pubs.niaaa.nih.gov
/publications/Practitioner/YouthGuide/YouthGuide.pdf.

69 *The American Academy of Pediatric:* https://www.aap.org/en-us/about
-the-aap/aap-press-room/pages/AAP-Recommends-Substance-Abuse
-Screening-as-Part-of-Routine-Adolescent-Care.aspx?nfstatus=401
&nftoken=00000000-0000-0000-0000-000000000000&nfstatus
description=ERROR:+No+local+token.

CHAPTER 5: MEANINGFUL
ENGAGEMENT AND ALTERNATIVES

73 *prime minister of Canada has now made heroin available:* http://www
.cnn.com/2016/09/14/health/prescription-heroin-canada/index
.html.

74 *the harms associated with drug use have decreased:* Hari, *Chasing the
Scream.*

76 *President Barack Obama wrote:* http://people.com/celebrity/roger
-ebert-remembered-by-president-obama-martin-scorsese/.

76 *Robert Redford described Ebert:* https://en.wikipedia.org/wiki/Roger
_Ebert.

76 *Oprah Winfrey remarked that his death:* Ibid.

76 *Steven Spielberg said that Ebert's:* https://www.theguardian.com/film
/2013/apr/05/roger-ebert-obama-spielberg-tributes.

76 *needed to leave some pretty big problems behind:* Roger Ebert, *Life Itself*
(New York: Grand Central Publishing, 2012).

80 *Mindfulness is yet another Eastern contribution:* K. Witkiewitz et al.,
"Mindfulness-Based Relapse Prevention for Substance Craving,"
Addictive Behaviors 38 (2013): 1563–71.

81 *Steve Jobs once said:* Walter Isaacson, *Steve Jobs* (New York: Simon &
Schuster, 2011).

82 *the subjects did not report distress:* M. Pollan, "The Trip Treatment,"
New Yorker, February 9, 2015; and M. C. Mithoefer et al., "Novel
Psychopharmacological Therapies for Psychiatric Disorders: Psilocy-
bin and MDMA," *Lancet Psychiatry* 3 (2016): 481–88.

82 *Their work identifies altered connectivity:* R. L. Carhart-Harris et al.,
"Neural Correlates of the LSD Experience Revealed by Multimodal

Neuroimaging," *Proceedings of the National Academy of Sciences* 113, no. 17 (2016): 4853–58.

83 *Some researchers even wonder about its beneficial effects:* C. S. Grob et al., "Pilot Study of Psilocybin for Treatment of Anxiety in Patients with Advanced-Stage Cancer," *Archives of General Psychiatry* 68, no. 1 (January 2011): 71–78.

83 *Ketamine has additionally been shown to have:* Michael H. Bloch et al., "Effects of Ketamine in Treatment-Refractory Obsessive-Compulsive Disorder," *Biological Psychiatry* 72, no. 11 (December 1, 2012): 964–70.

84 *the "meaningful engagement of talents":* Harvey B. Milkman and Stanley Sunderwirth, *Craving for Ecstasy* (San Francisco: Jossey-Bass, 1998).

84 *physical expression, self-focus, aesthetic discovery:* Kenneth W. Wanberg and Harvey B. Milkman, *Criminal Conduct and Substance Abuse Treatment: Strategies for Self-Improvement and Change: The Provider's Guide,* 2nd ed. (Thousand Oaks, CA: Sage Publications, 2008).

CHAPTER 6: PRINCIPLES OF TREATMENT

87 *an epidemic in the United States and other countries:* https://www.cdc.gov/drugoverdose/epidemic/.

88 *a comprehensive treatment plan for a person:* https://youtube.com/watch?v=QqnpkyCitx0.

93 *In my book for families: The Family Guide to Mental Health Care* (New York: W. W. Norton, 2013).

94 *No book on human behavior:* James O. Prochaska and Janice M. Prochaska, *Changing to Thrive* (Center City, MN: Hazelden Publishing, 2016).

95 *This is one area where doing less:* L. I. Sederer, *Improving Mental Health: Four Secrets in Plain Sight* (Arlington, VA: American Psychiatric Association Publishing, 2017).

97 *Dr. Pat Deegan was an originator:* https://www.patdeegan.com/.

98 *But he had developed trust and confidence:* Bruce Springsteen, *Born to Run* (New York: Simon & Schuster, 2016), 311–12.

NOTES

103 *With many individuals the methods which I employed:* Big Book, Alcoholics Anonymous, 26–27.

104 *cultural competence that can be adopted:* R. Lewis-Fernández et al., *DSM-5 Handbook on the Cultural Formulation Interview,* 1st ed. (Arlington, VA: American Psychiatric Association Publishing, 2016).

105 *Our behaviors, our habits—such as:* M. T. Compton and R. S. Shim, eds., *The Social Determinants of Mental Health* (Arlington, VA: American Psychiatric Association Publishing, 2015).

105 *Americans are prone to "mistaking health care for health":* P. Lantz et al., "Health Policy Approaches to Population Health," *Health Affairs* 26, no. 5 (2007): 1253–57.

107 *The occasion was a preview of an ESPN documentary:* Unguarded, directed by Jonathan Hock, ESPN, November 1, 2011. The full film is at https://vimeo.com/79305689.

108 *He tells his story with humility:* Adapted from L. I. Sederer, "*Unguarded*: The High Life of Chris Herren," *Huffington Post,* http://www.huffingtonpost.com/lloyd-i-sederer-md/chris-herren -addiction_b_1063575.html.

110 *Addiction is ubiquitous in our society:* To read more, including about Robin Williams and Philip Seymour Hoffman, go to http:// www.askdrlloyd.com/blog/view/humanmasks-and-mental-illness. For Prince's story, go to http://www.usnews.com/opinion/articles /2016-05-10/what-were-overlooking-about-opioids-pills-and -princes-death.

110 *Studies of AA estimate that it works for 5–10 percent:* Gabrielle Glaser, "The Irrationality of Alcoholics Anonymous," *Atlantic,* April 2015.

113 *Today, Patrick Kennedy has over six years:* Patrick J. Kennedy and Stephen Fried, *A Common Struggle* (New York: Blue Rider Press, 2015).

117 *It can be a desirable alternative:* http://www.smartrecovery.org/.

118 *This is not MI:* https://www.youtube.com/watch?v=80XyNE89eCs.

118 *The same doctor, with the same patient:* https://www.youtube.com /watch?v=URiKA7CKtfc.

118 *some critical first steps in managing:* A short video on MI can be found at https://www.youtube.com/watch?v=s3MCJZ7OGRk.

118 *William Miller, PhD, was a pioneer in MI:* Miller and Rollnick, *Motivational Interviewing.*

119 *Whatever may be your background:* A seventeen-minute video by a certified MI trainer puts it all together: *MI Skills Introduction*, https://www.youtube.com/watch?v=s3MCJZ7OGRk.

119 *Aaron T. Beck, MD, first popularized this creative approach:* Aaron T. Beck, *Cognitive Therapy and the Emotional Disorders* (New York: Plume, 1979).

120 *This approach began in the 1970s:* G. A. Marlatt and D. M. Donovan, *Relapse Prevention*, 2nd ed. (New York: Guilford, 2005).

120 *The US Substance Abuse and Mental Health Services Administration (SAMHSA):* SAMHSA Relapse Prevention, http://store.samhsa.gov/term/Relapse-Prevention.

127 *Community Reinforcement and Family Training (CRAFT):* J. Foote et al., *Beyond Addiction* (New York: Scribner, 2014), esp. pp. 7, 280–83.

127 *CRAFT is described by the American Psychological Association:* American Psychological Association, http://www.apa.org/pi/about/publications/caregivers/practice-settings/intervention/community-reinforcement.aspx. See also R. J. Meyers and B. L. Wolfe, *Get Your Loved One Sober: Alternatives to Nagging, Pleading, and Threatening* (Center City, MN: Hazelden Publishing, 2004).

127 *This approach benefits both the person:* Foote et al., *Beyond Addiction*, 7.

133 *Their best-known book, with Dr. Philip Muskin:* R. Brown, P. Gerbarg, and P. Muskin, *How to Use Herbs, Nutrients, and Yoga in Mental Health Care* (New York: W. W. Norton, 2012, paperback).

134 *Their even more recent book:* R. Brown, P. Gerbarg, and P. Muskin, *Complementary and Integrative Treatments in Psychiatric Practice* (Arlington, VA: American Psychiatric Association Publishing, 2017).

135 *As my good friend Dr. Drew Ramsey:* Drew Ramsey, *Eat Complete* (New York: Harper Wave, 2016).

142 *Drug courts are another useful policy intervention:* http://www.nadcp.org/learn/what-are-drug-courts.

142 *Drug courts work. Seventy-five percent of those:* Ibid.

145 *Addiction remains America's most neglected disease:* Adapted from L. I.

Sederer, "Addiction: The Equal Opportunity Threat to Life," *Huffington Post*, August 9, 2013.

CHAPTER 7: WHAT COMES NEXT

148 *Dr. Nora Volkow wrote in her inimitable way:* N. D. Volkow, G. F. Koob, and A. T. McLellan, "Neurobiological Advances from the Brain Disease Model of Addiction," *New England Journal of Medicine* 374, no. 4 (January 28, 2016).

149 *Eric Nestler, MD, at the Icahn School of Medicine:* E. J. Nestler, "Is There a Common Molecular Pathway for Addiction?," *Nature Neuroscience* 8 (2005): 1445–49, doi:10.1038/nn1578.

150 *A human vaccine study on people addicted:* https://nihrecord.nih.gov /newsletters/2015/08_14_2015/story2.htm.

151 *Deep brain stimulation (DBS), as well:* Helen Mayberg, "Neurologist Tests Deep Brain Stimulation to Relieve Depression," *NIH Record*, https://nihrecord.nih.gov/newsletters/2015/08_14_2015/story2.htm.

151 *Chronic stress fosters compromised immunity:* Sederer, *Improving Mental Health*.

153 *The work of my former colleague Dr. Roger Weiss:* R. D. Weiss et al., "Long-Term Outcomes from the National Drug Abuse Treatment Clinical Trials Network Prescription Opioid Addiction Treatment Study," *Drug and Alcohol Dependence* 150 (2015): 112–19.

154 *The use of long-acting naltrexone:* J. D. Lee et al., "Extended-Release Naltrexone to Prevent Opioid Relapse in Criminal Justice Offenders," *New England Journal of Medicine* 374, no. 13 (March 31, 2016).

CHAPTER 8: THE PAINTED BIRD

155 *A boy wanders about Eastern Europe:* Jerzy Kosinski, *The Painted Bird* (New York: Grove Press, 1965).

158 *"Hi, my name is Sam":* Joseph J. Bradley, *Addiction: From Suffering to Solution* (Breaux Press International, 2014), 99.

159 *MHPAEA supplements prior provisions:* https://www.dol.gov/ebsa /mentalhealthparity/.

159 *Championed by former congressman Patrick J. Kennedy:* L. I. Sederer,

"Mental Health and Civil Rights: The Kennedy Legacy," February 24, 2016, http://www.huffingtonpost.com/lloyd-i-sederer-md/mental -health-and-civil-rights-the-kennedy-legacy_b_9302968.html.

161 *BC2M seeks "to end the stigma"*: Bring Change 2 Mind, http://www .bringchange2mind.org/.

161 *A second effort is being led by the National Council:* http://www.the nationalcouncil.org/; and Mental Health First Aid, www.mentalhealth firstaid.org/.

161 *I WILL LISTEN is a third, powerful:* I WILL LISTEN, http://nami nyc.iwilllisten.org/.

162 *One poignant example, from her "10 Truths":* P. Lincourt, "10 Truths People with Substance Disorder Tell," *Huffington Post*, June 23, 2016, http://www.huffingtonpost.com/entry/10-truths-people-with -substance-disorder-tell_us_576ca4ebe4b06721d4c051b2.

APPENDIX: A BRIEF HISTORY OF OPIOID USE AND ABUSE IN AMERICA

176 *De Quincey wrote, "Happiness might now be bought":* Thomas De Quincey, *Confessions of an English Opium-Eater* (London: Crescent Press, 1950), 258.

176 *Laudanum and "black drop" opium:* John A. Renner, "Opioid Dependence in America," in *Handbook of Office-Based Buprenor- phine Treatment of Opioid Dependence*, by Petros Levounis and John Renner (Arlington, VA: American Psychiatric Association Publish- ing, 2011), 1.

176 *Their popularity was in part because doctors:* Lloyd Sederer, "Moral Therapy and the Problem of Morale," *American Journal of Psychiatry* 134, no. 3 (March 1977): 267.

176 *A panacea as powerful as opium:* Jones, *Hep-Cats, Narcs*, 18.

176 *Broadly utilized, it was reportedly:* Ibid., 17.

177 *In 1852, Scottish physician Alexander Wood:* https://www.general-anaes thesia.com/images/alexander-wood.html.

177 *Estimates are that four hundred thousand were addicted:* http://civilwar rx.blogspot.com/2016/06/soldiers-disease.html?_sm_au_=iVVrn2w Q2nFJV27M.

177 *The German word for this drug was* heroisch*:* Jones, *Hep-Cats, Narcs,* 36.

177 *In America that same year, a New York:* Morris Manges, *New York Medical Journal,* November 26, 1898, 768–70.

178 *By 1900 an estimated quarter million people:* Renner, "Opioid Dependence in America," 4.

179 *Epitomizing this shift, in 1903, Dr. George Pettey:* George Pettey, "The Heroin Habit: Another Curse," *Alabama Medical Journal,* 1903: 174–80.

179 *The Pure Food and Drug Act paved:* Musto, *Drugs in America,* 26–31.

179 *The State Department drove its passage:* Jones, *Hep-Cats, Narcs,* 40–41.

180 *In addition, over three thousand physicians were jailed:* Martin Booth, *Opium: A History* (New York: St. Martin's Griffin, 1996).

180 *By the 1920s, thanks to the Harrison Act:* Jones, *Hep-Cats, Narcs,* 57.

181 *By the decades after World War II:* https://www.samhsa.gov/data/sites/default/files/NSDUH-DetTabs-2015/NSDUH-DetTabs-2015/NSDUH-DetTabs-2015.pdf.

181 *Annual estimates of its use became available:* Martins et al., "Changes in US Lifetime Heroin Use."

181 *One report indicated a tenfold increase:* Booth, *Opium,* 204.

181 *In the 1960s, at the Rockefeller Institute in New York:* Jones, *Hep-Cats, Narcs,* 287–94.

182 *But its use has always been limited:* Renner, "Opioid Dependence in America," 21.

182 *A review of its history suggests that for many years:* Jones, *Hep-Cats, Narcs,* 297.

183 *By 1994, this war had led:* http://content.time.com/time/magazine/article/0,9171,962371-1,00.html; https://web.stanford.edu/class/e297c/poverty_prejudice/paradox/htele.html; and https://www.vera.org/.

183 *While far fewer veterans persisted in their addiction:* Zinberg, "Heroin Use in Vietnam and the US," 486–88.

183 *These reports became the basis of a vast marketing campaign:* Charlestown Gazette Mail, http://www.wvgazettemail.com/news-health/20161217/drug-firms-poured-780m-painkillers-into-wv-amid-rise-of-over doses.

184 *But once it was in place, doctors had:* http://americanpainsociety.org/uploads/education/section_2.pdf.

184 *The CDC has recently become active:* http://www.usnews.com/news /blogs/data-mine/2015/08/19/the-heroin-epidemic-in-9-graphs.

185 *Heroin use has increased more among men:* "Death Rates Rising for Middle-Aged White Americans," https://www.nytimes.com/2015/11 /03/health/death-rates-rising-for-middle-aged-white-americans-study -finds.html?_r=0.

185 *This has been understood, in part, as a result:* National Employment Law Project, "The Low Wage Recovery: Industry Employment and Wages Four Years into the Recovery" (New York, 2014).

185 *In 2002, introduced by federal legislation called DATA 2000:* Renner, "Opioid Dependence in America," 20.

187 *As previously noted, by 2013, opioid sales:* https://www.cdc.gov/nchs /products/databriefs/.

INDEX

fight-or-flight response, 78, 151, 152, 153, 169
Fitzgerald, F. Scott, 156
folic acid, 92, 169
"follow the money" (control strategy), 49–50
Food and Drug Administration (FDA), 83, 179, 181–82
Ford Foundation, 18
Freud, Anna, 35
Freud, Sigmund, 35, 152
friends
    and principles of good treatment, 94, 101, 104, 105, 107
    research about, 153
    resources for, 145
    See also peers; relationships

GABA receptors, 149
gambling: as compulsive behavior, 3
Ganguly, Shruti, 48
gender: and history of addiction, 185
genetics
    and challenges concerning addiction, 146
    and factors influencing addiction, 14
    and principles of good treatment, 105
    research about, 150, 154
Gerbarg, Patricia, 133–34
glutamate, 83, 132–33, 134, 140, 149
Gold, Samuel (pseud.), 99–101
Gomez, Luisa (ACE example), 62–63
Graciela (ACE example), 64–66
group therapy
    as treatment program, 120–21
    See also specific group

half-life
    definition of, 23–24
    as factor influencing addiction, 23–25
hallucinogens. See psychedelic drugs; specific drug
Halsted, William Stewart, 12–13, 20

Hammelsmith, Charlie "Chaz," 76
Hari, Johann, 14, 74
harm-reduction strategies
    and factors influencing addiction, 20–21
    and treatment for addictions, 136–40
Harrison Narcotics Tax Act (1914), 179–80
hashish, 23
Health and Human Services Department, US (HHS), 70, 159
hepatitis C, 21, 136
heroin
    and agonists, 130
    availability of, 185
    as big culprit of addiction, x
    and brain, 186
    cost of, xi
    criminalization/illegalization of, 45, 180
    deaths from, x, 187
    epidemic of, 6, 7, 180
    and factors influencing addiction, 15, 18–19
    and fail-first policies, 45
    and history of addiction, 6, 7, 177–78, 180, 181, 182, 183, 184–85
    importation of, 180
    legalization of, 73
    and Man with a Golden Arm, The (film), ix, 119
    medical professional views about, 180
    overdosing on, 7, 184, 185, 187
    perspectives about, 87
    and perspectives about treatment, 90
    popularity/prevalence of, 2, 4, 180, 181, 183, 184
    and prescription drug monitoring programs, 142
    and principles of good treatment, 107–9
    and race/class, 184
    treatments for, 5, 130, 181, 182
    and vaccines, 149
Herren, Chris (patient), 107–9

ABOUT THE AUTHOR

Lloyd I. Sederer, MD, has published a dozen books and more than five hundred articles in the fields of mental health and the addictions as well as film, TV, theater, and book reviews. He is an adjunct professor at the Columbia University Mailman School of Public Health and the chief medical officer for the New York State Office of Mental Health, the nation's largest state mental health agency. He is also a monthly regular on *Tell Me Everything*, the Sirius XM radio show hosted by John Fugelsang. His recent books include *Improving Mental Health: Four Secrets in Plain Sight* and *Current Controversies in Mental Health and Addictions*.

Dr. Sederer has received numerous psychiatric and medical awards, including the Irma Bland Award for Excellence in Teaching Residents by the American Psychiatric Association, a scholar-in-residence grant by the Rockefeller Foundation, and an Exemplary Psychiatrist Award from the National Alliance on Mental Illness. As the chief medical officer for the New York State Office of Mental Health, he oversees the care of more than seven hundred thousand individuals annually and the operations of mental health clinics and hospitals throughout the state. Previously, Dr. Sederer served as the executive deputy commissioner for Mental Hygiene Services in New York City (the NYC mental health commissioner); medical director and executive vice presi-

ABOUT THE AUTHOR

dent of McLean Hospital in Belmont, Massachusetts, a Harvard teaching hospital; and director of the Division of Clinical Services for the American Psychiatric Association.

Dr. Sederer has contributed articles to dozens of publications, including both medical journals and mainstream outlets such as the *New York Times/International New York Times*, the *Wall Street Journal*, the *Washington Post*, *Commonweal* magazine, and *Psychology Today*. A leader in the field of the addictions and mental health care, he has been practicing medicine for more than forty years.